CONTENTS

INTRODUCTION

Inflammation is your immune system's response to injury or unwanted microbes in your body. It is a natural process and vital part of your body's healing process. When inflammation becomes systemic and chronic, however, it becomes a problem, and measures need to be taken. This type of inflammation serves no purpose, and can cause a lot of harm to the body.

As a nutritionist, I have clients suffering from a wide spectrum of health issues, and inflammation is easily one of the most common issues. Some of these clients are in constant pain, often excruciating. Migraines are a regular occurrence, and they don't sleep too well either. Their energy reserves always seem depleted and even sleep doesn't help, even if they manage to get a few good hours in.

I always suggest these clients to get a blood test for C-reactive protein if they haven't got one already, and if you feel you suffer from any symptoms of inflammation, I suggest you go to a nearby lab and get this blood test done right away. Chances are that your C-reactive protein levels are higher than normal, and the best way to manage this is diet. Shouldn't be hard though, considering how delicious anti-inflammatory foods are! Even if you do not suffer from chronic and systemic inflammation, incorporating anti-inflammatory foods in your diet will be one of the best decisions you will make in your life. You will notice the difference when you start. Your energy levels will be much higher, your mood will be uplifted, and you will feel more alive, in general.

This book has a LOT of recipes, and not every recipe might work for you. For example, if you're allergic to dairy or gluten, the recipes containing those ingredients will cause more harm than good. However, substitutions are possible for all of these, so you will be fine following this book as long as you keep an eye on the ingredients and use a bit of creativity where you have to! Once you understand the fundamentals of the diet, you will be fully equipped to create your own recipes from scratch!

In this book, you will learn all about the ingredients that are alleviate inflammation, and those that aggravate it, so you can make an educated guess for what's the best recipe for you, and what's the worst, even if you're out eating at a restaurant.

Causes Of Chronic Inflammation

Medical science is striving to pinpoint the causes of chronic inflammation, and according to the Autoimmunity Research Foundation, numerous possible causes have been identified. This knowledge has mainly been derived from observational studies in which researchers can find correlation, though correlation does not equate to causation. Which is to say that while causes are identified by the studies, there is no scientifically proven concrete link between causes and outcomes. This uncertainty is an integral part of epidemiological studies, but they can still provide some very useful information.

Suggested causes for widespread chronic inflammation include:

- Antibiotic overuse and misuse (including in the food supply and through prescribed medications)
- Dietary factors (processed foods, unbalanced essential fatty acids, and chemical additives, among others)
- Environmental factors (endocrine disrupters and pesticides, among others)
- Use of substances (medications) that suppress immune responses, such as anti-inflammatories, antibacterial agents, and corticosteroids

In addition, Medical News Today (MNT) notes other factors that may play a role in chronic inflammation, including:

- Autoimmune diseases
- Obesity
- Poor sleep quality and sleep deprivation

Chronic Inflammatory Diseases

The research goes on but quite a few diseases have been linked to chronic inflammation. In this section, we will take a look at some of these.

Autoinflammatory Disease

According to the National Institutes of Health's (NIH) National Institute of Arthritis and Musculoskeletal and Skin Diseases (NIAMS), autoinflammatory disease is a rather new class that is quite unlike autoimmune disease, although the names are rather similar and they share some features. Autoimmune diseases are caused by the immune system attacking healthy tissue, leading to chronic inflammation. The reason for this is not fully understood by science just yet.

Autoinflammatory diseases can cause intense, chronic inflammation that can lead to symptoms such as fever and joint swelling. A few common diseases in this category are:

- Behçet's disease
- Chronic Atypical Neutrophilic Dermatosis with Lipodystrophy and Elevated Temperature (CANDLE)
- Deficiency of the Interleuken-1 Receptor Agonist (DIRA)
- Familial Mediterranean Fever (FMF)
- Neonatal Onset Multisystem Inflammatory Disease (NOMID)
- Tumor Necrosis Factor Receptor-Associated Periodic Syndrome (TRAP)

Autoimmune Disease

NIAMS says that autoimmune diseases also have a chronic inflammatory component to them. When your body sees its own healthy tissue as an intruder, it attacks it. Inflammation is one of the key signs of autoimmune disease, although, depending on the disease, other symptoms might be exhibited too.

More than 80 autoimmune diseases have been identified at the time of writing this book, and some of the most common ones are listed below:

- Addison's disease
- Ankylosing spondylitis

- Celiac disease
- Crohn's disease
- Endometriosis
- Fibromyalgia
- Grave's disease
- Hashimoto's disease
- Interstitial cystitis
- Juvenile (type 1) diabetes
- Juvenile arthritis
- Lupus
- Lyme disease (chronic)
- Multiple sclerosis
- Psoriasis
- Rheumatoid arthritis
- Scleroderma
- Ulcerative colitis
- Vitiligo

Cardiovascular Disease

The American Heart Association notes that while it isn't currently established that inflammation causes cardiovascular disease (diseases of the heart and blood vessels), it is usually present, particularly in arteries of people suffering from this kind of a disease. Multiple factors are associated with heart disease, such as tobacco use, high blood pressure, and high levels of "bad" cholesterol called low-density lipoprotein (LDL), etc., so managing these is key to preventing and managing cardiovascular diseases.

Type 2 Diabetes And Obesity

An article in the May 2, 2005 issue of the Journal of Clinical Investigation studied the link between type 2 (adult onset) diabetes, inflammation, and stress, and found a close correlation between inflammation and type 2 diabetes, mostly triggered by obesity. This research suggests that obesity activates multiple chemical responses in the body that result in extensive inflammation, and this inflammation further causes metabolic disorders like type 2 diabetes.

Managing Chronic Inflammation

With advances in medical science, we have quite a few options for managing chronic inflammation. Some of the most popular options today are as follows.

Nsaids

Nonsteroidal anti-inflammatory drugs (NSAIDs) such as ibuprofen or naproxen sodium (Aleve) are often recommended by health experts for managing and treating inflammation. However, these can potentially cause side effects, especially when used in the long term.

Corticosteroids

These synthetic steroids are administered both orally and externally, and are great at suppressing the body's immune response. However, these too can cause side effects in the long run.

Herbal Remedies

Minor inflammation can be managed by simple herbal remedies containing anti-inflammatory ingredients like turmeric and ginger. Combining turmeric with black pepper, coconut oil, or quercetin increases its bioavailability, thus making it easier for the body to absorb it.

Lifestyle Changes

Simple lifestyle changes such as exercise, yoga, meditation, better sleep, losing weight, stress reduction techniques, etc. can go a long way in managing inflammation.

Anti-Inflammatory Diet

The anti-inflammatory diet is a fairly new concept, and research is still going on. However, a review in the December 2010 issue of Nutrition in Clinical Practice notes an anti-inflammatory eating pattern which balances the ratio of essential fatty acids (omega-3 to omega-6 fatty acids) and consists mainly of fresh fruits, vegetables, legumes, and whole grains while reducing saturated fats (such as fats from meat) and maximizing monounsaturated fats (such as olive oil), is much better at managing inflammation than a typical western diet.

Anti-Inflammatory Eating Habits

You are what you eat. Eat good, look good, feel good. Eat trash, look like trash, feel like trash.

Fighting Inflammation Through Diet

The anti-inflammatory diet has a very simple concept. When you plan your meals, you maximize the ingredients that reduce inflammation, and minimize/eliminate the ingredients that aggravate inflammation. Though, this is easier said than done.

We live in a world where everything, even food, is available at the flick of your finger. We are surrounded by delicious processed food with chemical additives, preservatives, and unhealthy fats. When such good taste comes with such high convenience, it is easy to give in.

However, if you do manage to overcome your urges, and decide to eat healthy, I'll tell you what you need to look for. Head to a nearby farmers' market and pick out fresh anti-inflammatory ingredients. Some of the most potent anti-inflammatory ingredients are listed under the next heading.

Anti-Inflammatory Ingredients

Not all ingredients are created equal when it comes to the anti-inflammatory diet. Some are simply better and more potent than the others. I am a woman of science, and medical research has revealed some of the best ingredients for managing inflammation. If you're serious about this diet, you will do well to have all these ingredients on hand at all times.

Bell Peppers

Bell peppers—particularly red bell peppers—are a great source of antioxidants and capsaicin, both of which are exceptional at fighting inflammation. Add them to recipes containing turmeric for an anti-inflammatory bomb. They also contain quercetin, which enhances your body's absorption of anti-inflammatory curcumin. Be careful using these if you're sensitive to nightshades though.

Broccoli

High in fiber and immunity-boosting antioxidants like vitamin C, broccoli is a potent inti-inflammatory ingredient.

Kale

This vegetable is loaded with fiber and antioxidants.

Spinach

Loaded with antioxidants like vitamin C and K, spinach is great at fighting inflammation.

Tomatoes

As long as you're not sensitive to nightshades, tomato is amazing at fighting inflammation, thanks to the lycopene contained within.

Blueberries

Blueberries are rich in antioxidants, and augment your immune system while fighting inflammation. Oh, and they taste absolutely amazing!

Salmon And Other Fatty Fish

A good balance of essential fatty acids (omega-3 and omega-6 fatty acids) is absolutely vital to combat inflammation. Omega-3 fatty acids are anti-inflammatory, while omega-6 fatty acids are pro-inflammatory. Functional medicine specialist Chris Kresser notes that the perfect ratio of omega-6 fatty acids to omega-3 fatty acids is 1:1 or 2:1. The problem with the typical western diet is that this ratio is really unbalanced. The omega-6 fatty acid is so high in the western diet that the ratio can be as bad as 25:1!

To counter this, supplemental fish oil rich in omega-3 fatty acids can be taken, or better yet, a diet rich in salmon and other fatty fish can be taken. These fish taste absolutely amazing, and are great anti-inflammatory ingredients!

Nuts

Nuts rich in omega-3 fatty acids are best. Some of these are: walnuts, cashews, almonds, pecans, etc. These have a high calorie density, so eat in moderation if you're looking to lose weight.

Cinnamon

Cinnamon contains cinnamaldehyde, which, according to an article in the January 2008 issue of Food and Chemical Toxicology, is a great at fighting inflammation.

Garlic

One of the most potent anti-inflammatory ingredients, garlic has been used in home remedies since ancient times. Modern science too has now confirmed that garlic enhances the immune system, and is one of the best anti-inflammatory ingredients out there.

Ginger

Ginger adds an amazing flavor to whichever dish it is added, and boasts potent anti-inflammatory properties to boot!

Rosemary

This fragrant and flavorful herb is a potent anti-inflammatory ingredient. It goes especially well in a non-vegetarian dish.

Turmeric

Turmeric contains curcumin, which many studies have concluded is great at fighting inflammation.

Extra-Virgin Olive Oil

EVOO is loaded with healthy fats, and contains oleocanthal, which is a potent anti-inflammatory compound.

Green Tea

Green tea is loaded with antioxidants, enhances the immune system, and has anti-inflammatory properties.

Ingredients To Watch Out For

While a certain ingredient might reduce inflammation in one person, it might do the exact opposite for another. Below is the list of a few ingredients that are common allergens, and if a certain recipe in this book doesn't help with inflammation, try eliminating these ingredients first.

The anti-inflammatory diet for every person will be a little different, and you are the only person who can find what ingredients suit you best. Below is the list of ingredients to watch out for:

- Dairy Products: A lot of people are allergic to casein, whey, and lactose. All three are contained in milk, and if you're allergic to even one of these, substitute dairy for nondairy alternatives such as almond milk or hemp milk.
- Eggs: This is an allergen that is hard to substitute in most cases. If you're baking, eggs can be replaced by flax eggs. Flax eggs can be made by mixing 1 tbsp ground flaxseed with 2½ tablespoons water and allowing to rest for 5 minutes until thick. This substitutes one egg in baking recipes.
- Fish: If you're allergic to fish, try shellfish instead. If you're allergic to that too, try chicken instead. Try tofu in fish recipes for a vegan dish. Soy sauce is a great alternative to fish sauce.
- Gluten: Gluten is one of the most common allergens out there. This protein is found in wheat, barley, etc. Two of my favorite gluten free grains are millet and quinoa.
- Nightshades: If you're sensitive to these, you should avoid eating tomatoes, tomatillos, goji berries, eggplant, bell peppers, chile peppers, and potatoes. Two alternatives are onions are garlic, but nightshades can never truly be substituted.
- Peanuts: Peanut allergy is quite common. It is a legume so substitute it with a nut you like and are not allergic to.
- Soy: If you're allergic to soy, you will need to read labels of all food items you buy. Tofu can be substituted by chicken, while soy sauce can be replaced by a spice blend of your choice.
- Tree Nuts: Tree such as almonds, walnuts, pecans, cashews, Brazil nuts, macadamia nuts, etc. are allergens to some. Try peanuts or a different nut you're not allergic to instead.
- Wheat: Another common allergen, wheat is easily replaced by buckwheat or rice flour.

Chapter One

WHAT IS AN ANTI INFLAMMATORY DIET?

*P*ut simply, anti-inflammatory nutrition is a diet that has a positive effect on inflammation in the body. It helps to reduce existing inflammation and prevent new sources of inflammation from developing. Thus, an anti-inflammatory diet is much more than just a healthy diet in the traditional sense. If you manage to change your current diet accordingly, you could reduce the inflammation in your body, which promotes rheumatism in the joints, a little and thus reduce your symptoms in the long term.

From the point of view of nutritionists, the so-called Nutri-Epi (genetics) is still a very young research area. It deals with the effects of the constituents of our food on protein production in the body and on the changes in metabolism that can result from this protein production. Scientists already assume that we can influence inflammation in the body with the natural components of food. For example, the ingredients of plants have in some cases been examined quite well. Ingredients such as resveratrol from red grapes or raspberries, catechins from green tea, bioflavonoids or polyphenols from coffee have already been researched quite well. They are said to have a good anti-inflammatory effect, so an appropriate diet should always consist of plenty of fruit and vegetables. In the opinion of many nutritionists, an anti-inflammatory diet is very similar to the well-known Mediterranean cuisine, which only had to be modified slightly. Legumes, herbs, lettuce, fruit, nuts, fish and little meat are part of such a diet. If you are on an anti-inflammatory diet, be careful not to use olive oil. Rapeseed oil can be used as a substitute. You should also remove foods with simple carbohydrates from your menu, although bread, pasta or rice in the whole grain variants are entirely permitted and suitable.

The healthy basis of your diet consists of vegetables, high-quality protein in the form of nuts with legumes and high-quality oils such as wheat germ oil or linseed oil. When it comes to fruit, you should make sure that it does not contain too much sugar. The consumption of oil should of course be limited due to its high calorie content. However, you can supplement a muesli for breakfast with a splash or two of oil, so the ingredients, vitamins and minerals in fruit, for example, come into their own. You can also enrich a smoothie with vegetables in this way; if you add a little oil, the vitamins are even better absorbed and processed by the body. Switching to a low-fat diet is of great importance to an anti-inflammatory diet. Nutritionists assume that a diet high in unhealthy fats promotes inflammation in the body. They are triggered by very complex biochemical metabolic processes. Mediators that trigger certain reactions in the immune system are involved in the inflammation. These promote the development of inflammation. If you manage to switch to an exclusively vegetarian diet, you could significantly alleviate many typical rheumatoid symptoms such as lack of mobility in the morning or swollen joints. This is because with a vegetarian diet, on the one hand, you consume less harmful fatty acids, but on the other hand, you also consume healthy fatty acids. If you don't want to go without meat in your anti-inflammatory diet, that's not a problem, as long as you stick to one or two servings a week.

The interplay of fatty acids in an anti-inflammatory diet is also interesting. As you already know, arachidonic acid is one of the most important causes of inflammation in the body. This fatty acid has several opponents, which are also found in fatty acids. Omega-3 fatty acids from vegetable oil or fish prevent the conversion of the harmful arachidonic acid into the pro-inflammatory mediators and promote the formation of anti-inflammatory acids in the body. This means that they have a direct effect on the inflammation foci in the joints. Eicosapentaenoic acid has proven to be very effective. This omega-3 fatty acid is found in oily fish such as salmon, tuna or herring. Alpha-linolenic acid also has a very anti-inflammatory effect; it occurs in vegetable oils, with rapeseed, soy or walnut oil being preferred. Fish oil preparations are said to have a very positive effect on the inflammatory processes in the body. However, it is important that you always discuss the use of such products as a dietary supplement with your doctor. You should only follow an anti-inflammatory diet after consulting him so that he can adjust your medication accordingly. In this way you prevent the unwanted and uncontrolled ingestion of anti-inflammatory drugs and foods and, overall, arrive at a coherent therapy that will bring you the greatest benefit.

The intake of antioxidants also has a positive effect on inflammation in the body. Free radicals are aggressive in the body and promote inflammation. Antioxidants counteract this inflammation, thereby rendering the aggressive oxygen radicals almost harmless. Vitamins E and C, but also beta-carotene or trace elements such as copper, selenium or zinc prove to be good catchers of free radicals. Since these vitamins and minerals are ingested through fruits and vegetables, it is clear why you should ensure that they are adequate. You now know that an anti-inflammatory diet can be very beneficial to your wellbeing. Give it a try and change your diet for a period of time. Try how you are feeling and whether you have the impression that your symptoms are getting better. Even if you start out with just one or two measures at first because you are having a hard time switching to a full anti-inflammatory diet, stick to it and don't give up too soon. The best effect is achieved by a complete change in diet, in which you observe all individual steps and implement them to the full. It should be noted, however, that there are hardly any scientific or medical studies that prove the influence of a changed diet on rheumatism. While nutritionists believe there is a link, long-lasting medical studies are still rare. This is all the more true for long-term studies that could prove a change in the processes in the body in the long term.

Even in the absence of such studies, you can get a pretty good idea of how you are doing after changing your diet. Observe yourself and your body and closely monitor symptoms. Check how the morning stiffness of your joints is developing and when and how often inflammation or pain attacks occur. Pay attention to your body and the symptoms, especially if they are getting better or worse. You will then get a good sense of whether or not your anti-inflammatory diet is working well or not. You can continue to support your body by changing your drinking habits. In order for the biochemical processes in the body to function properly, you must provide it with sufficient water and fluids. With a weight of around 60 kilograms, a woman should drink around 1.8 liters a day, a man of 80 kilograms should drink around 2.4 liters. Make sure that it is water or tea. Liquids with a high content of sugar, coffee or even alcohol are not drinks that are well tolerated by the body and that support its functions. On the contrary, if you overdo it, alcohol is known to have very harmful effects on the body. Only the very moderate consumption of red wine can have a positive effect on your rheumatism. Regardless of the intensity with which you change your diet, there is one more aspect that you should not lose sight of. The time horizon plays a major role. Nutritionists believe it will take at least three months for the body to adjust to the new diet and for the first effects to appear. So be patient if you want to change your diet so that your rheumatism improves. This is particularly difficult with frequent pain attacks, and many patients then tend to get impatient. However, there is little point in eating a healthy diet for a few weeks only to break one or the other bad habit. Make an effort to stick to your anti-inflammatory diet as consistently as possible and stay consistent for at least three months. It is even better if you can take it longer and eat healthy and balanced food for at least a year. Your body then has the best chance of getting used to the new form of nutrition, so that the biochemical processes in the body gradually change. However, if you manage to get your rheumatism under control step by step, the incentive should be enough to stick to a healthy and anti-inflammatory diet, whereby one or the other small sin is of course allowed. For example, if you've caught yourself sinful once, enjoy it and resume your healthy diet the next day. In any case, this is better than overdoing it in the sense of "all or not at all" and then going back to the old unhealthy diet.

What else can you do for your body?

Anyone who is plagued by regular rheumatism attacks is probably also wondering what else can be done, apart from diet, to relieve and support the body. In principle, the most important recommendations can be summarized in a single sentence: Strive for an all-round healthy lifestyle. You can find out what is particularly important in this section.

Put cigarettes aside!

This tip is certainly not surprising. Rheumatoid smokers shouldn't be surprised if they have to take more and stronger drugs than non-smokers. In general, smokers have a greater risk of developing rheumatism. Every cigarette favors the development of chronic inflammatory processes in the body. The only way to avoid this is to put the cigarette packet to one side and not touch any more cigarettes. The result speaks for itself, however, because with every non-smoked cigarette you increase your quality of life.

Drink alcohol only in moderation!

Alcohol is like cigarettes. It is harmful to your body. With every glass of beer, wine, sparkling wine and the like, you weaken the body's own defense processes and stress your immune system. This directly affects the sensitive anti-inflammatory processes in the body. Of course, a small glass of red wine occasionally does no harm, but in your own interest as a rheumatoid patient you should definitely forget about regular consumption of alcohol.

Exercise!

The third tip is certainly not unfamiliar to you either. With regular exercise, you ensure that your joints and tendons remain fit and flexible. Whether you start with physiotherapy, whether you sign up for the gym or whether you regularly put on your running shoes is up to you. Choose a sport that you enjoy, because only then will you stick with it. Incidentally, it is very healthy for your bones if you get some fresh air every day. It doesn't matter if the sky is overcast or if the sun is shining. Movement is good for you, and even light rays of the sun support the body in producing the important vitamin D. Vitamin D ensures that the calcium from food is transported into your body and into the bones, where it can act against inflammation.

Relax!

In our hectic everyday life between work and family, it is often not easy to remain calm and relaxed. However, stress has a direct effect on inflammation in the body, because it ensures that the production of free radicals in the body increases. If you are a rheumatoid patient, you should avoid this at all costs, because free radicals cause inflammation in the body to skyrocket. That is why regular relaxation and adequate sleep are two very important criteria for you and your body to be well. Even if it is often very difficult in everyday life not to stress and overwhelm yourself, you should definitely take this tip seriously. It may also help you learn a relaxation technique that you can use right away if needed.

Take care of your oral hygiene!

This recommendation may sound surprising. However, bacteria settle in the mouth and throat, and especially in the gums, which can trigger your immune system. At first there is inflammation in the gums, but in the worst case also an infection of the bone that lies underneath. Medical studies have shown that there is a connection between such inflammation and rheumatic inflammation in the body. You should therefore take care of your teeth and gums and visit your dentist regularly so that he can prevent any inflammation in the mouth and throat at an early stage.

You now know how you can contribute a lot to your well-being with the right diet and a healthy lifestyle, even if you as a rheumatoid patient are dependent on regular medication. Your doctor is sure to provide you with the best all-round medication, and you can do a lot to help keep yourself well. If you make an effort to follow an anti-inflammatory diet and adopt a sensible lifestyle, you will win back the most beautiful gift that you should not underestimate, even with a chronic illness: a high quality of life that makes life worth living in old age.

BREAKFAST: BLUEBERRY QUINOA

Ingredients for 2 people:
1/2 teaspoon vanilla extract
50 g raisins
1 cup of quinoa
1 teaspoon cinnamon powder
1 small apple, cut into cubes
750 ml unsweetened almond milk
1 cup blueberries (alternatively raspberries or strawberries)
1 handful of sunflower seeds
Apple syrup
1 handful of walnuts

PREPARATION:

First, put the quinoa in a saucepan with the almond milk and cinnamon. After that, everything is brought to a boil. As soon as the contents boil, the pot is covered. Now the stove is put on a low flame so that the contents simmer gently. Stir everything well from time to time so that nothing burns. After everything has simmered again for 5 minutes, the apple cubes and the raisins are added. Then everything has to simmer again for 5 minutes. After the 5 minutes have elapsed, the pot is removed from the stove so that the contents can be drawn with the lid closed. Now everything is seasoned with the apple syrup and the berries and nuts are stirred in. Then the blueberry quinoa can be served.

MUESLI WITH CRUNCH: INGREDIENTS FOR 2 PEOPLE:

2 dates
2 ripe bananas
Juice of half a lemon
2 apples
1 tbsp agave syrup
4 teaspoons of tiger nuts
6 walnut halves

PREPARATION:

First the bananas and apples are peeled. The bananas are then cut into slices and the apples into small pieces. The cut fruit is put aside in a bowl. The dates are also cut into small pieces and the walnut halves roughly chopped. Now the roughly chopped walnut halves are placed in a coated pan with the agave syrup and briefly roasted. Then the walnut halves are mixed into the fruit together with the tiger nut flakes, lemon juice and dates.

THE FRUITY BOMB: INGREDIENTS FOR 2 PEOPLE:

1/2 pineapple
1 pear
2 kiwis
2 carrots

Preparation:

The pineapple is peeled and cut into pieces. The pieces should fit in a juicer later. The carrots are brushed with a vegetable brush under running water and also cut into pieces for the juicer. Likewise, the kiwi is peeled and cut into pieces if necessary. The pear is washed and pitted thoroughly. Then it is cut into coarse cutlets. Now the fruit juice is pressed with the juicer. Fill this into a glass and enjoy the fruity bomb.

PORRIDGE WITH TIGER NUTS: INGREDIENTS FOR 1 PERSON:

1 teaspoon of crushed flaxseed
4 tbsp organic tiger nut flakes
2 dried, unsulphurized figs
100 ml hot spring water (alternatively hot almond milk)
1/2 apple
1 banana

PREPARATION:

The tiger nut flakes are poured over with hot water, stirred and set aside to swell. In the meantime, the banana can be peeled and mashed with a fork. The apple is washed and finely grated. The figs are also cut into small pieces. Finally, the mashed bananas, the grated apple and the figs are added to the tiger nut flake porridge together with the flaxseed. For serving, the porridge is arranged in a bowl.

PORRIDGE WITH APPLE: INGREDIENTS FOR 1 SERVING:

cardamom
3 tbsp buckwheat
1 apple
2 tbsp oatmeal
cinnamon
2 tbsp almonds
unsweetened grain drink (oats, almonds or spelled)

PREPARATION:

The almonds are roughly chopped and soaked in a little water with the buckwheat overnight and then rinsed through a sieve the next day. The almonds and buckwheat are now put in a saucepan with the grain drink and oat flakes. Everything is heated on a low flame with the pot closed. In the meantime, the apple is grated and can be added to the

porridge. Finally, season everything with cardamom and cinnamon and
serve warm.

PORRIDGE WITH COCONUT AND RASPBERRIES: INGREDIENTS FOR 2 PEOPLE:

salt
150 g raspberries
6 tbsp oatmeal
150 g red currants
350 ml coconut milk
50 g desiccated coconut
1 tbsp rice syrup

PREPARATION:

First the good raspberries and currants are sorted out. After that, they are
washed, carefully patted dry and placed in a bowl. Now the raspberries
and currants are mixed together and set aside. The coconut milk is put in
a saucepan with the oat flakes, desiccated coconut and a pinch of
salt. Bring everything to the boil while stirring. Then the porridge is taken
off the stove to cool down. For serving, the porridge is layered alternately
with the berry mixture in a glass. If you want, you can garnish everything
with mint leaves.

GINGER AND CUCUMBER SMOOTHIE: INGREDIENTS FOR 1 SERVING:

1 tbsp linseed oil
1/2 cucumber
2 handfuls of lamb's lettuce
Water ad libitum
2–3 tart apples
1 piece of ginger, finger length
1 handful of romaine lettuce

PREPARATION:

First the fruit, the cucumber and the lettuce leaves are washed. The apples are then quartered and pitted. The ginger is roughly chopped. All ingredients are then placed in a tall vessel and pureed with a hand blender or stand mixer.

OMELETTE WITH TOMATO: INGREDIENTS FOR 2 PEOPLE:

2 tbsp rapeseed oil
1 shallot
salt and pepper
100 g feta
2 tbsp mineral water
2 dried tomatoes
3 eggs
2 fresh tomatoes

PREPARATION:

The shallot is peeled and diced. The feta is crumbled and the dried tomatoes are cut into fine slices. The fresh tomatoes are washed, halved and pitted. Then they are cut into fine cubes. Now the eggs are whisked with salt, pepper and the mineral water. The oil is heated in a pan and the shallots are fried until golden. Then add the egg mixture and sprinkle with the crumbled feta and tomatoes. The egg must now set on a mild heat. Then the finished omelette can be halved and served on two plates.

NETTLE SEED LOW-FAT CURD: INGREDIENTS FOR 1 SERVING:

1 tbsp nettle seeds
1 tbsp wheat germ oil
75 g blueberries (fresh or frozen)
1 teaspoon rose hip powder
200 g low-fat quark

1 pinch of turmeric
1 tbsp flaxseed
1 tbsp linseed oil

PREPARATION:

The blueberries are rinsed and patted dry. Frozen blueberries must be thawed beforehand. The low-fat quark is stirred with the oil until smooth. The mixture can be made creamier with a little water if the oil is not enough as a liquid. The turmeric, rose hip powder and nettle seeds are now mixed into the low-fat quark. The blueberries are poured over it for serving.

OMELETTE WITH SMOKED SALMON: INGREDIENTS FOR 2 PEOPLE:

2 tbsp rapeseed oil
300 g cucumber
2 tbsp chives rolls
salt and pepper
2 tbsp dill, freshly chopped
1 box of garden cress
2 tbsp kefir
50 g smoked salmon
2 tbsp mineral water
3 eggs

PREPARATION:

The cucumbers are washed or peeled and cut diagonally into thin slices. Then the cucumber slices are laid out flat on a plate and sprinkled with salt. The salmon is cut into cubes and set aside. The cress is cut from the bed, washed and patted dry. The eggs are now whisked with salt, pepper, mineral water and the kefir. The dill and chives are lifted under the egg mixture. The oil is heated in a pan and the egg mixture is added. On low heat, the egg mixture must now set to an omelette. The diced salmon and cress are sprinkled over the omelette in the pan. This is now folded up, halved and served on the prepared cucumber slices on the plate. The finished omelette can be served immediately.

BANANA AND NUT MASH: INGREDIENTS FOR 1 SERVING:

1 tbsp linseed oil
30 g tiger nut flakes
30 ml coconut milk
1 banana
80 ml cashew milk

Preparation:

First mash the banana. Then mix in the tiger nuts flakes. Mix the whole thing with the coconut milk and cashew milk. Finally stir in the linseed oil.

APPLE AND NUT MUESLI: INGREDIENTS FOR 1 SERVING:

1 cup of lupine yogurt
1 apple
1 tbsp pumpkin seeds
2 tbsp tiger nut flakes
4 almonds
2 walnuts

Preparation:

Wash and dice the apple. Chop the walnuts and almonds. Mix both with the apple. Roast the pumpkin seeds in a pan without fat and add them to the apple. Then mix in the tiger nuts flakes. Finally, stir the whole thing with the lupine yoghurt.

FRUIT BOWL: INGREDIENTS FOR 1 SERVING:

2 tbsp hemp flour
1 avocado
1 banana
1 green apple

Preparation:

Halve the avocado and remove the stone. Puree the pulp of the avocado together with the banana. Then add the hemp flour and stir. Dice the apple and add it. Mix everything again.

APRICOT QUINOA PORRIDGE: INGREDIENTS FOR 3 SERVINGS:

1 tbsp pumpkin seeds
100 g quinoa
300 ml of oat milk
6 apricots

Preparation:

First wash and drain the quinoa. Bring the oat milk to the boil and cook the quinoa in it for about 10 minutes. In the meantime cut the apricots in half and remove the stones. Puree the pulp of the apricots. Put the finished quinoa in a bowl and mix with the pureed apricots. Finally, chop the pumpkin seeds and roast them in a pan without fat. Sprinkle these over the apricot quinoa porridge.

TIGERNUT PORRIDGE: INGREDIENTS FOR 1 SERVING:

1 pinch of cinnamon
60 g tiger nut flakes
1 teaspoon raw cocoa
100 ml rice milk

Preparation:

Bring the rice milk to the boil and stir in the tiger nuts flakes. Let the whole thing swell for about 10 minutes. Finally, season with the cocoa and cinnamon.

QUINOA PORRIDGE WITH CHERRIES: INGREDIENTS FOR 2 SERVINGS:

1 tbsp agave syrup
100 g quinoa
300 ml lupine drink
50 g frozen cherries

Preparation:

Bring the lupine drink to the boil in a saucepan. Then add the quinoa and simmer over medium heat for about 10 minutes. Then take the saucepan off the stove and add the frozen cherries. Finally, season the whole thing with the agave syrup.

ALMOND PANCAKES: INGREDIENTS FOR 1 SERVING:

Coconut oil
50 g almond flour
2 teaspoons coconut blossom sugar
20 g coconut flour
2 tbsp almond butter
20 g raw cocoa
200 ml almond milk

PREPARATION:

Mix the cocoa with the two types of flour. Then add the coconut blossom sugar and the almond milk and stir well. Heat the coconut oil in a pan and fry the dough in portions to make pancakes. Brush the finished pancakes with the almond butter.

RASPBERRY AND ALMOND MASH: INGREDIENTS FOR 1 SERVING:

1 teaspoon coconut blossom sugar
75 g quinoa
1 tbsp almond slicer
20 g ground almonds
50 ml of oat cream
50 g frozen raspberries
200 ml rice drink

PREPARATION:

Heat the rice drink in a saucepan. Let the quinoa simmer in it for about 10 minutes. Then stir in the ground almonds, oat cream and coconut blossom sugar. Let the whole thing swell briefly. Finally fold in the frozen raspberries and garnish with the almond slices.

NUT AND FRUIT MUESLI: INGREDIENTS FOR 1 SERVING:

1 cup of lupine yogurt
10 g of popped amaranth
10 g unsweetened banana chips
10g popped quinoa
10 g dried apples
10 g chopped almonds
10 g chopped walnuts

PREPARATION:

Mix all ingredients together except for the yoghurt. Finally add the yoghurt and stir everything together.

VEGETABLE AND FRUIT SMOOTHIE: INGREDIENTS FOR 1 SERVING:

1 teaspoon coconut blossom sugar
1 pear
100 ml almond milk
1 carrot

Preparation:

Peel and halve the pear. Then remove the core housing. Dice the carrot. Put the pear and carrot in a blender and puree. Then add the almond milk and mix everything again. Season the smoothie with the coconut blossom sugar.

FRUIT YOGURT DRINK: INGREDIENTS:

1 tbsp coconut butter
1 banana

100 g lupine yogurt
50 g sour cherries
100 ml rice drink

Preparation:

Peel and cut the banana. Core the cherries and remove the stems. Put both in a blender and puree. Then add the rice drink and coconut butter and mix again. Finally add the yoghurt.

ORANGE SMOOTHIE: INGREDIENTS:

250 ml almond milk
1 peach
4 apricots

Preparation:

Wash the fruit and cut in half. Remove the stones and seeds. Then puree the fruit and add the almond milk. Mix the whole thing well together again.

ALMOND AND FRUIT SMOOTHIE: INGREDIENTS:

1 teaspoon almond butter
1 apple
100 ml almond milk
100 g sweet cherries

Preparation:

Wash the fruit and remove the stones and stems. Cut the apple into small pieces and puree with the cherries. Then add the almond milk and almond butter and mix everything together again.

YEAST-FREE SPELLED BREAD: INGREDIENTS FOR 1 BREAD:

olive oil
500 g spelled flour (type 630)
100 g pumpkin seeds
1/2 teaspoon salt
100 g of flaxseed

500 ml of lukewarm water
1 pk. Tartar baking powder
1 teaspoon bread spice mix

PREPARATION:

Mix the baking powder with the flour. Then mix in the bread spices, flax seeds and pumpkin seeds. Then add the water and knead everything together. Brush a loaf pan with the olive oil and pour in the batter. Then brush the surface of the dough again with a little water. Bake the bread for 60 minutes at 200 ° C top / bottom heat.

FRUIT PULP WITH POMEGRANATE SEEDS: INGREDIENTS FOR 2 SERVINGS:

1 pomegranate
100 g buckwheat
100 ml almond milk
2 pears
2 teaspoons of lemon juice
1 banana
2 tsp almond butter
1 apple
2 teaspoons of sweet lupine flour as required
1 handful of raisins

PREPARATION:

Soak the buckwheat in water for 1 hour. Then pour through a sieve and rinse. So that the buckwheat can germinate, place the sieve over a bowl and rinse under water in the morning and evening. As soon as the buckwheat sprouts, place 3–4 tablespoons on a baking sheet and leave to dry in the oven at 50 ° C for approx. 3–4 hours. Put the remaining buckwheat with the flour, lemon juice, raisins and almond butter and almond milk in a blender. Remove the core from the apple and pears. Cut all the fruit into small pieces and add to the buckwheat mixture. Mix everything well. If the porridge is too firm, it can be diluted with a little almond milk. Remove the seeds from the pomegranate. Put the finished porridge in a bowl and spread the pomegranate seeds and the cooled buckwheat kernels on top.

FRUIT CEREAL: INGREDIENTS FOR 1 SERVING:

2–3 tbsp oat flakes (alternatively granola)
1 small banana
some blueberries
1 tart apple
1 juice orange

PREPARATION:

First squeeze the orange. Cut the banana into slices and mix carefully with the orange juice. Wash the apple and cut into small cubes. Mix the apple with the blueberries into the banana. Finally fold in the oatmeal.

FRUIT PORRIDGE: INGREDIENTS FOR 1 SERVING:

1 handful of fresh fruit (alternatively dried fruit)
3–4 tablespoons of glued oat flakes
1 teaspoon chopped almonds
100 ml coconut milk
1 teaspoon sesame seeds
1 pinch of salt

PREPARATION:

Heat the coconut milk and stir in the oatmeal. Then simmer the porridge for about 3–5 minutes over low heat. Remove the pan from the heat and season the porridge with the salt. Cut the fruit into small pieces and fold into the pulp.

BANANA MASH: INGREDIENTS FOR 1 SERVING:

Vanilla or cinnamon
300 ml almond milk
1 banana
4 tbsp ground tiger nuts
2 tbsp lupine protein vanilla

PREPARATION:

In a saucepan, bring the almond milk with the lupine protein and the tiger nuts to the boil. Let it simmer for 5–7 minutes. During this time, mash the banana. Fold the mashed banana into the pulp. Finally, season the whole thing with vanilla or cinnamon.

APRICOT AND CINNAMON PORRIDGE: INGREDIENTS FOR 2 SERVINGS:

1 pinch of salt
120 g millet
1/3 teaspoon cinnamon
150 ml coconut milk
2 tbsp ground flaxseed
200 ml of water
1 tbsp sesame seeds
1 apple
2 tbsp coconut flakes
4 dried, unsulphurized apricots

PREPARATION:

First wash and rinse the millet. Bring the coconut milk, water, sesame, linseed, millet and salt to the boil. In the meantime, wash the apple and remove the core. Cut the pulp into pieces and add to the coconut milk. Chop the apricots and stir in. Let it simmer over a low heat for 5–6 minutes. Then put everything aside for about 10 minutes to swell. Toast the coconut flakes in a pan without oil. Finally fold in the coconut flakes and cinnamon.

GREEN VEGETABLE SMOOTHIE: INGREDIENTS FOR 1 SERVING:

6–8 ice cubes
1 avocado
1 pk. Stevia
1/2 English cucumber
1 teaspoon of super green powder
1 small tomato
2 teaspoons of bean sprouts powder
1 lime
2 cups of fresh spinach

PREPARATION:: FIRST PEEL THE LIME. HALVE THE AVOCADO AND REMOVE THE STONE. PUT EVERYTHING IN A BLENDER AND MIX.

Spicy smoothie
Ingredients:
Ice cubes
1 small cucumber
1 pinch of salt and pepper
1 stick of celery
1/2 chilli pepper
4 Roma tomatoes
1 lemon (alternatively 2 limes)

PREPARATION:

Cut the vegetables into small pieces and puree them in a blender. Squeeze the juice from the lemon and add to the vegetables. Chop the chilli pepper and add it along with salt and pepper. Mix everything again. Fill ice cubes in glasses and distribute the smoothie in them.

VEGETABLE JUICE: INGREDIENTS:

3 carrots
1 medium-sized cucumber
1 medium beetroot
1 green pepper
2 tomatoes

Preparation:

Cut the vegetables into small pieces and squeeze out the juice with a juicer. The vegetable juice can be diluted with water.

VEGETABLE AND MINT SMOOTHIE: INGREDIENTS FOR 1 SERVING:

2-3 mint leaves
2 carrots
3 ice cubes
1 grapefruit
100 ml of pure water

Preparation:

Peel the carrots and grapefruit. Put both in a blender and puree. Dilute the smoothie with the water and add the mint leaves.

TOFU SMOOTHIE WITH VEGETABLES: INGREDIENTS:

3-4 ice cubes
1 avocado
unsweetened soy milk
1 lime
1 handful of fresh spinach leaves
1 small cucumber

PREPARATION:

Halve the avocado and remove the stone. Then peel the avocado and lime. Cut the pulp of both into pieces. Cut the cucumber and tofu into cubes. Put everything in a blender and puree.

COCONUT FRUIT MUESLI: INGREDIENTS FOR 1 SERVING:

1 tbsp flaxseed
1 peach
1 tbsp quinoa sprouts
1 mandarin
30 g coconut flakes
Preparation:

Rinse the quinoa sprouts and flax seeds. Mix the coconut flakes with the almond milk. Wash and core the peach. Peel the tangerine. Cut this and the peach into small pieces. Finally mix everything together.

FRUIT MUESLI WITH CINNAMON: INGREDIENTS FOR 1 SERVING:

1 teaspoon carob powder
50 g fresh papaya
1 pinch of cinnamon
50 g fresh avocado
1 tbsp Chufas nuts
1 soaked fig
1-2 teaspoons acerola powder
1 soaked date
2-3 teaspoons of spirulina powder
1 small banana

PREPARATION:

Soak the dried fruits, then puree them with the soaking water, spirulina powder, carob powder, papaya and cinnamon. Put the Chufas nuts in a bowl and pour the dried fruit puree over it. Mix everything together well. Cut the banana into slices and sprinkle with the acerola powder. Finally mix everything again.

LEEKS: INGREDIENTS FOR 1 SERVING:

1 pinch of crystal salt
100 g tender leeks
1 pinch of miso
30 g buckwheat groats
5 g sunflower oil
8–10 tbsp vegetable broth without yeast (alternatively water)

PREPARATION:

Put the groats in boiling water while stirring and let swell over low heat. In the meantime, finely chop the leek and steam in a little water. Then mix the leek into the buckwheat groats and remove everything from the stove. Finally, season to taste with the oil, miso, vegetable stock and salt.

COLORFUL BREAKFAST PORRIDGE: INGREDIENTS FOR 1 SERVING:

some raisins or dried fruit
1 carrot
Walnuts as needed
1 apple
1 banana

Preparation:

Peel the carrot and apple. Remove the core from the apple. Cut the pulp of the apple, the carrot and the banana into large pieces. Puree all ingredients together.

PLUM SMOOTHIE WITH WALNUTS: INGREDIENTS FOR 2 SERVINGS:

250 ml of water
8 plums
40 ml of cherry juice
300 ml of water
4 teaspoons of flaxseed

1 banana
12 walnuts

PREPARATION:: SOAK THE PLUMS IN THE WATER. THEN PUREE ALL INGREDIENTS TOGETHER.

Main courses
Millet pancakes
Ingredients for 2–3 people:
Sea salt or organic salt
500 g millet
50 g sesame seeds
1 small carrot (alternatively 1/2 medium-sized carrot)
50 g sunflower seeds
1 1/2 onions
1 tbsp gluten-free soy flour
extra virgin, cold-pressed olive oil

PREPARATION:

Cut the onions and the carrot into small cubes. Put half a diced onion together with the carrot, millet and 1 teaspoon sea salt in 2 liters of water. Let everything simmer for about 40 minutes. Then put the cooked millet in a bowl and add the remaining onion that has already been diced. Also add the soy flour, sunflower seeds, sesame seeds and 1/2 teaspoon sea salt and mix everything together well. Now form a buffer from this. Heat some olive oil in a pan and gradually fry the buffers in it.

SAVOY CABBAGE POTATO PAN: INGREDIENTS FOR 4 PERSONS:

Vegetable broth
1 savoy cabbage
3 cloves of garlic
turmeric
1 red pepper
1 onion
1 large carrot

cumin
6 potatoes

PREPARATION:

The thick parts of the stalk are removed from the savoy cabbage leaves. The leaves are divided and then cut into strips. These are blanched in boiling salted water for 3 minutes. Dice the onion, potatoes, carrots and peppers and fry them in a pan with the flat-pounded garlic. Now deglaze the whole thing with 1/2 cup of water and steam with the lid closed for 5 minutes. After the 5 minutes have passed, add the savoy cabbage and season with vegetable stock, cumin and turmeric to taste. Mix everything together well and steam again for 5–10 minutes. It should be stirred again and again. If desired, sunflower seeds or pumpkin seeds can be added on top.

PASTA WITH ZUCCHINI AND EGGPLANT: INGREDIENTS FOR 2–3 PEOPLE:

Sea salt and freshly ground black pepper
300 g spelled pasta
2 tsp basil leaves, dried
1 large, diced aubergine (approx. 300 g)
1 teaspoon oregano
3 tbsp extra virgin olive oil
2/3 cup vegetable broth
1–2 finely diced, medium-sized onions
4 tbsp dried, diced tomatoes
3 medium, ripe, diced tomatoes
1 large, diced zucchini (approx. 400 g)

PREPARATION:

Heat the olive oil in a large pan. Fry the onions, garlic and aubergines for 8–10 minutes, stirring occasionally. Then the zucchini and all the tomatoes with the oregano are added and cooked again for 6–8 minutes. In between, the mass should be stirred so that nothing burns.

In the meantime, the spelled pasta is cooked al dente in water. Then the vegetable stock is added to the pan and everything is seasoned with salt, pepper and the dried basil. Let the pan simmer for a few minutes. To serve, the finished sauce is poured over the pasta.

VEGETABLE CURRY: INGREDIENTS FOR 2 SERVINGS:

Sea salt and fresh pepper
200 g carrots
1 tsp curry powder
250 g broccoli florets
100 ml of yeast-free vegetable stock
100 g peas
100 ml unsweetened coconut milk
1 tbsp oil
1 clove of garlic
1 medium onion

PREPARATION:

Chop the onion and garlic and set aside. The carrots are cut into slices and also set aside. In a pan or wok, heat the oil over a medium flame and sauté the onions, garlic and curry powder until translucent. Then add the carrot slices and broccoli florets and stir briefly. Then coconut milk and vegetable broth are added and everything is simmered on a low flame for 8-10 minutes with the lid closed. Every now and then everything should be stirred. Finally, season the whole thing with pepper, sea salt and a little lemon juice (if necessary). Bring everything to the boil again briefly and then serve.

RATATOUILLE: INGREDIENTS FOR 4 SERVINGS:

1 cup of water
5 tomatoes
1 pinch of cayenne pepper
1 large zucchini

1 pinch of sea salt (or organic salt)
1 large eggplant
3 tablespoons of cold-pressed, extra virgin olive oil
1 green pepper
2 tsp herbs from Provence (basil, marjoram, lavender, thyme, oregano, rosemary, sage)
1 large onion
2 cloves of garlic

PREPARATION:

The skin is removed from the peppers and tomatoes and the pulp is cut into cubes. The eggplant, onion, zucchini and garlic are cut into thin slices.
Put some olive oil in a pan or wok and heat. Sauté the onions and garlic for a few minutes. Then the zucchini slices, the diced paprika and the aubergine slices are added and sautéed for another 10 minutes. Occasionally everything should be stirred. Then the tomatoes, herbs and water are added and everything is mixed together well. Let it simmer again for a few minutes. Finally, the whole thing is seasoned with salt and pepper.

GREEK LENTIL SOUP: INGREDIENTS FOR 4 SERVINGS:

1/2 teaspoon oregano
300 g small, Greek lentils
1 bay leaf
2 fresh tomatoes
Sea salt and fresh pepper
1 carrot
1 tbsp fresh lemon juice
1/2 stick of leek
2 tablespoons of cold-pressed, extra virgin olive oil
1 onion
3-4 cloves of garlic

PREPARATION:

The lentils are washed well and soaked in plenty of water overnight. Drain the lentils the next day and simmer in hot water for 5 minutes. Then the lenses are poured off and drained again. The onion and cloves of garlic are finely chopped. Pureed the tomatoes and cut the carrots and leek into fine slices. Now put the tomato puree, the carrot slices, the onions, the chopped garlic cloves and the leek slices together with the bay leaf in 1/2 liter of water and bring to the boil over high heat. Then add the lentils and simmer gently over low heat for at least 30 minutes. It may be necessary to add some water. Finally, the olive oil and lemon juice are added and everything is seasoned with oregano, sea salt and pepper.

CELERY BROCCOLI SOUP: INGREDIENTS 2 SERVINGS:

salt and pepper
1 onion
0.5–1 liters of almond milk
1 head of celery
1–2 liters of vegetable stock
1 broccoli
Spices of your choice to taste
1 teaspoon oil

PREPARATION:

Chop the onion and fry in a little oil in a large stock pot for about 5 minutes. Cut the celery into pieces and set aside some of the leaves for garnish. Also cut the broccoli into small pieces and put in a blender along with the celery. Mix both ingredients until the vegetables are finely chopped. Add the celery and broccoli mix to the onions and heat. Then add the vegetable stock and the almond milk and simmer for about 15-30 minutes. Then puree the entire contents of the pot until a fine, creamy consistency is achieved. At the end everything is seasoned with salt and spices of your choice. The soup can be served warm or cold.

CHICKPEA SALAD WITH AVOCADO: INGREDIENTS FOR 2 PEOPLE:

3 spring onions
1 can of chickpeas
1 red pepper
1 handful of fresh spinach leaves
100 g asparagus (fresh or from the jar)
1 romaine lettuce
1 stick of celery
3 tomatoes
For the dressing:
1 pinch of sea salt
1 avocado
extra virgin, cold-pressed olive oil
Juice of one lemon

PREPARATION:

Except for the avocado, all ingredients are cut into small pieces and placed in a salad bowl. Then everything is mixed together well. Cut the flesh of the avocado into small pieces and place in a blender with the lemon juice and a little olive oil. Mix everything briefly until you have a thick dressing. If the dressing becomes too thick, a little water can be added. Pour the finished avocado salad dressing over the salad with a pinch of salt and mix everything together well.

STUFFED PEPPERS: INGREDIENTS FOR 2 SERVINGS:

sea-salt
1 large bell pepper (red or yellow)
1 large, ripe avocado
7 medium, fresh carrots
fresh herbs to taste

PREPARATION:

First, the peppers are washed, cut in half and both halves thoroughly cleaned. Then they can be put aside. The carrots are pressed through a juicer and processed into juicy pulp. Then the avocado is peeled and the pulp is pressed into the carrot puree with a fork. The carrot and avocado puree can now be seasoned with sea salt and the fresh herbs. At the end it is filled into the pepper halves and can be served.

AVOCADO SOUP: INGREDIENTS FOR 1 SERVING:

some water
1 avocado
1 pinch of sea salt
1 stick of celery
1 pinch of pepper
1 splash of fresh lemon juice
1 handful of fresh spinach
1 tomato

PREPARATION:

First the tomato is cut into small cubes. Then all the other ingredients are put in a blender and mashed on high. The finished soup can now be put in a soup bowl. Add the diced tomatoes and serve.

POTATO SALAD: INGREDIENTS FOR 4 PERSONS:

Salt and white pepper
1 kg of potatoes
3 tbsp oil
1/8 liter stock (instant)
1 bunch of radishes
4 tbsp herb vinegar
1 small stick of leek

PREPARATION:

First the potatoes are washed and then cooked for 20 minutes. Then the water is poured off and the potatoes can be peeled and put aside to cool. Once the potatoes have cooled, they are quartered and cut into pieces. Now pour the hot broth over the potato pieces and let it steep for 10 minutes. In the meantime, mix the herb vinegar, salt and pepper into a marinade. The potatoes are now mixed with the marinade. The whole thing now has to go through well again. Meanwhile, the leek is cleaned, washed and cut into fine rings. The radishes are also cleaned, washed and cut into fine slices. Before the potato salad is served, the radishes and leek are mixed with the oil with the salad.

VEGETABLE PAN WITH GARLIC DIP: INGREDIENTS FOR 2 PEOPLE:

For the pan:
Iodized salt and pepper
4 spring onions
fresh or dried herbs (oregano, thyme, rosemary)
2 carrots
1 tbsp olive oil
1 small zucchini
1 red pepper
For the dip:
Iodized salt and pepper
1 cup of yogurt, 1.5% fat
1 clove of garlic
2 tbsp sour cream
1 tbsp olive oil

PREPARATION:

First the vegetables are cleaned, washed and cut into fine strips. The olive oil is heated in a coated pan and the vegetables are added. Now the vegetables are cooked firm to the bite for about 15 minutes over medium heat and often turned. Finally, the vegetable pan is seasoned with iodized salt, pepper and the herbs.

For the dip:

Mix the yoghurt with the sour cream and the olive oil. The garlic clove is squeezed out and also added. Finally, season the dip with salt and pepper.

SWISS CHARD LASAGNA: INGREDIENTS FOR 10-12 PEOPLE:

500 g of grated cheese
2.5 kg of Swiss chard
2.5 liters of vegetable stock
625 g mushrooms
7 tbsp flour
500 g onions
7 tbsp butter
1000 g lasagne sheets
7 tbsp oil

PREPARATION:

First the chard is cleaned and the green leaves are removed from the stems. The stems are cut into short strips and the leaves are roughly chopped. Everything is blanched in a saucepan with boiling water and then drained. The mushrooms are cleaned and sliced. The onions are diced and sweated in oil. Now the mushrooms and the chard are added. With the lid closed, everything is steamed for about 10 minutes. The butter is melted and the flour is stirred in. The whole thing is extinguished with the vegetable stock and briefly boiled. Now the sauce is seasoned. Finally, the vegetables, the sauce and the lasagne sheets are layered alternately in a baking dish. First the sauce and the last layer must also be sauce. Sprinkle the lasagne with the grated cheese and bake at 170 ° C for 40 minutes.

BEETROOT SOUP: INGREDIENTS FOR 4 PERSONS:

salt

500 g beetroot
100 ml cream
1 onion
grated peel of an orange
2 carrots
750 ml vegetable stock
100 g potatoes
about 1 cm of ginger

PREPARATION:

First the beetroot and the onion are peeled and then diced. The carrots and potatoes are brushed and also cut into cubes. The ginger is peeled and grated. Sweat the onion cubes in oil and add the beetroot, carrots and potatoes. The ginger is then added and everything is topped up with the vegetable stock. Now the whole thing has to simmer for about 15 minutes. After the 15 minutes have elapsed, the contents of the pan are pureed. Now everything has to be seasoned with salt and the grated orange peel. Finally, the cream is whipped and drawn into the soup before serving. As an alternative: Instead of ginger and orange peel, you can also use some apple juice.

LIGHT PEA SOUP: INGREDIENTS FOR 4 PERSONS:

Salt and white pepper
2 pk. frozen peas (300 g each)
1/2 cup of whipped cream (100 g)
1 1/4 liters of clear broth
3 bunch of chervil / 3 eggs

PREPARATION:

Bring the peas together with the broth to the boil in a saucepan and cook for about 15 minutes. Then the peas are finely pureed with the cutting stick of the hand mixer. The eggs are placed in boiling water and hard-boiled for 10 minutes, after which they are peeled off, cut in half and the egg whites finely chopped. The chervil are washed thoroughly under running water and carefully shaken dry. Then some stalks are set aside and the rest are finely chopped. The egg white and chervil are added to the soup. Then the soup is seasoned with salt and pepper. The cream is slept stiffly and half drawn under the soup. The rest of the cream is given as a dollop on top of the soup for garnish. The egg yolk is now pressed through a fine press, for example a garlic press, and sprinkled over the soup together with the chervil that was set aside. Then the finished soup can be served.

CARROT SALAD WITH PINEAPPLE: INGREDIENTS FOR 2 PEOPLE:

4 large leaves of lettuce / 500 g carrots
2 tbsp coconut flakes / 2 slices of pineapple
1 tbsp raisins
For the marinade: 1 pinch of cayenne pepper
3 tbsp lemon juice / 1 pinch of ground coriander
3 tbsp pineapple juice / 2 tbsp oil / 1 tbsp honey

PREPARATION:

First the carrots are finely grated. The pineapple is cut into small cubes and the raisins are washed. Everything is mixed together with the coconut flakes. For the marinade: Mix the lemon juice with the pineapple juice and honey. Then everything is seasoned with the cayenne pepper and the coriander and oil is added. The marinade is now mixed with the salad and placed in a cool place so that the salad can permeate well. Before serving, the salad should be seasoned again. For serving, the plates are covered with the lettuce leaves and the carrot salad is served on top.

BAKED CAULIFLOWER: INGREDIENTS FOR 4 PERSONS:

1 cup of crème fraîche, 1.5 fat (150 g)
2 small heads of cauliflower
2 egg yolks
salt

1/2 teaspoon ground nutmeg
Fat for the shape
1 pk. Peas (300 g)
1 tsp curry
30 g butter or margarine
1/2 liter of almond milk
30 grams of flour

PREPARATION:

The cauliflower is cleaned, washed and cut into small florets. Then the florets are blanched for 5 minutes in boiling salted water. 1/2 liter of the cauliflower water is poured off through a sieve and stored. Put the cauliflower florets and the peas in a greased baking dish. Fat is heated for the sauce. The flour is sweated in it and then extinguished with the almond milk and the cauliflower water. Now the whole thing has to boil again, the sauce is seasoned with salt, curry and nutmeg. The egg yolk is mixed with the crème fraîche and stirred into the sauce. This is now poured over the vegetables in the baking dish and baked for 35-40 minutes at 200 ° C (electric stove). On a gas stove, the casserole is baked on level 3. If you want, you can serve mashed potatoes with it.

ZUCCHINI STEW: INGREDIENTS FOR 3 PEOPLE:

pepper from the grinder
40 g margarine
1/8 liter of water
2 onions
1 pinch of saffron
300 g zucchini
1 teaspoon oregano
1 small savoy cabbage
2 teaspoons of herbal salt
1 leek
50 g grated Gouda cheese
250 g tomatoes

PREPARATION:

Peel the onions and cut into rings. Steam the onion rings in a pan with fat until translucent. Cut the zucchini into slices, the savoy cabbage into strips and the leek into rings. Then the vegetables are added to the onions and sautéed briefly. Now the water is added and everything is cooked for 20 minutes. In the meantime, peel the tomatoes, cut them in half and add them to the pan after 10 minutes. In addition, everything is seasoned with herbal salt, pepper, saffron and oregano. Just before the dish is served, sprinkle everything with cheese and parsley. Crispy farmer's bread can be served with it.

CELERY AND APPLE RAW VEGETABLES: INGREDIENTS FOR 4 PERSONS:

1 tbsp chopped hazelnuts
250 g celeriac
1 lettuce
250 g sour apples
4 teaspoons of lemon juice
1 cup of skimmed milk yogurt (175 g)

PREPARATION:

Wash and then peel the celery and apples. The apples are quartered and pitted. The celery is cut into pieces. Then both ingredients are grated and immediately drizzled with lemon juice. The skimmed milk yogurt is stirred until smooth. The lettuce is washed, drained and the leaves are distributed on four plates. Spread the raw vegetables on the lettuce leaves and put a blob of yogurt per serving on top. The hazelnut kernels are then sprinkled over the top.

PEA SOUP WITH DUMPLINGS: INGREDIENTS FOR 4 PERSONS:

1/2 teaspoon salt
2 kg of fresh green peas

grated nutmeg
2 onions
1 bunch of parsley
75 g margarine
2 eggs
4 tbsp chicken broth
125 g spelled flour
1/4 liter of milk

PREPARATION:

The peas are first peeled, rinsed and drained. Now the onions are peeled and finely diced. Approx. Heat 50 g of the margarine and sauté the onions until translucent. Now the peas are added and steamed for 3 minutes. Now the chicken broth is sprinkled in and extinguished with 1.5 liters of boiling water. Let the soup simmer for 15 minutes. Now the milk, the salt and the rest of the margarine are brought to the boil in a saucepan. The flour is poured in and everything is stirred until it loosens from the bottom of the pot as a lump. Now the pot is removed from the stove and the eggs are gradually stirred into the batter. Now everything is seasoned. Small dumplings are cut from the dough and carefully added to the soup. These have to steep in the soup for 10 minutes. After that, everything is sprinkled with chopped parsley.

HERBSOUP: INGREDIENTS FOR 4 PERSONS:

a few drops of lemon juice
50 g margarine
nutmeg
2 tbsp spelled flour
1 liter of almond milk
1 bunch each of chives, parsley, dill
3 teaspoons of condensed milk

PREPARATION:

First the margarine is heated in a saucepan. Then stir in the flour and sweat it until it has a golden yellow color. The almond milk is now poured on while stirring. Everything is left to cook for a few minutes. The herbs are finely chopped in the meantime. One half of the chopped herbs is added to the milk mass. This is also seasoned with, nutmeg and salt. The herb soup is now boiled until it has a creamy consistency. Then it is seasoned again and the remaining herbs and condensed milk are stirred in. Finally, the finished soup is seasoned with lemon juice.

COLESLAW: INGREDIENTS FOR 1 BOWL:

1 pinch of cayenne pepper
1/2 cabbage
1 cup coconut milk (preferably fresh coconut meat mixed with the coconut juice)
2 medium-sized carrots
2 tbsp extra virgin olive oil
1 small, red onion
1/2 tbsp fresh lemon juice
1/2 cup parsley
1/2 teaspoon sea salt

PREPARATION:

The parsley is finely chopped. The cabbage, carrots and onion are cut into fine strips. All ingredients are put in a bowl and mixed well there. The coconut milk is now spread over the salad and also mixed well with the other ingredients. The finished salad must now pull through well.

KALE SALAD: INGREDIENTS FOR 2 SERVINGS:

a bit of salt
250 g kale

2 tbsp lemon juice
200 g edamame
4 tbsp virgin olive oil
75 g dried cranberries
100 g cherry tomatoes

PREPARATION:

First wash the kale, remove the stem and shake dry. Then pluck the kale into bite-sized pieces. Mix the olive oil with the lemon juice and the salt and mix the kale with it. Let the whole thing stand in the refrigerator for about 10 minutes. In the meantime, bring the salted water to the boil and simmer the edamame for 3–4 minutes until soft. Then drain and rinse with cold water. Wash the cherry tomatoes and cut in half. Mix the kale with the tomatoes, edamame and cranberries and season the salad with salt and pepper.

CURRY POTATO PAN: INGREDIENTS FOR 2 PEOPLE:

2 tbsp sesame seeds
400 g potatoes
salt and pepper
400 g pointed cabbage
1/2 can of coconut milk
1 bell pepper
1 tsp curry
2 carrots
2 teaspoons of turmeric
2 tablespoons oil
2 onions

PREPARATION:

First wash the pointed cabbage and remove the stalk. Then cut the cabbage into fine strips. Cut the onions into fine cubes. Peel, wash and dice the potatoes and carrots. Wash, core and cut the peppers into strips. Heat the oil in a pan and fry the onions, potatoes and carrots in it for about 10 minutes. Then add the cabbage and fry everything for about 3 minutes. Deglaze the whole thing with the coconut milk and season with the spices. Bring everything to the boil and arrange on plates. Sprinkle the potato pan with the sesame seeds.

DUMPLINGS: INGREDIENTS FOR 2 PEOPLE:

nutmeg
6 potatoes
White pepper
4 sprigs of parsley
Seasoned Salt
3 teaspoons of virgin olive oil

Preparation:

Wash, peel and cut the potatoes. Cook the potato pieces in a steamer for about 15–20 minutes. In the meantime, wash the parsley and gently shake dry. Then pluck the leaves from the parsley and chop finely. Mash the finished potatoes into a pulp and mix with the olive oil, salt, nutmeg, pepper and parsley. Form dumplings from the mixture with two tablespoons and arrange them on plates.

POTATO AND KOHLRABI SOUP: INGREDIENTS FOR 2 PEOPLE:

parsley
5 kohlrabi
pimento
2 potatoes
White pepper
1 shallot
grated nutmeg
3 tbsp sunflower oil
Seasoned Salt
750 ml of water
1 teaspoon gluten- and yeast-free vegetable broth without glutamate

PREPARATION:

Wash and peel the potatoes and kohlrabi. Then cut the kohlrabi into pieces. Finely chop the potatoes and shallot. Heat the oil in a saucepan. Sauté the shallots in it. Then add the potatoes and kohlrabi and let everything simmer for another 2 minutes. Deglaze everything with the water and the vegetable stock and bring everything to a boil. Cook the soup for another 15-20 minutes. Then season everything with the spices and puree. Wash and finely chop the parsley and sprinkle over the soup.

KOHLRABI AND CARROT SOUP: INGREDIENTS FOR 4 SERVINGS:

200 g kohlrabi / 400 g carrots
salt and pepper
40 g onions
1 tsp curry
10 g ginger
150 ml coconut milk
1 small chilli pepper
600 ml vegetable stock
20 g butter
Coriander green
some coconut milk

PREPARATION:

Peel the onion and carrots. Roll both dice. Peel and finely chop the ginger. Halve, core and finely chop the chilli pepper. Melt the butter in a saucepan. Steam the chilli, carrots, ginger and onion in it. Deglaze everything with the coconut milk and vegetable stock. Season the whole thing with the spices and simmer for 20 minutes over low heat. In the meantime, wash, peel and dice the kohlrabi. Puree the finished soup and add the kohlrabi cubes. Let everything simmer again for 8 minutes. Garnish the soup with the coriander greens and coconut milk before serving.

STRAWBERRY SALAD: INGREDIENTS FOR 4 SERVINGS:

For the salad:
1 teaspoon red pepper berries
400 g strawberries
12 basil leaves
100 g rocket
For the dressing:
2 tbsp grape seed oil
2 tbsp Balsamico Bianco / 1 pinch of stevia
salt and pepper

PREPARATION:

Wash the strawberries and remove the greens. Then drain and cut into slices. Wash the rocket too and remove the stalks. Spread both together with the basil on plates. Mix all ingredients for the dressing together and pour over the salad. Garnish with the pepper berries.

LAMB'S LETTUCE WITH MUSHROOMS: INGREDIENTS:

2 tbsp sunflower seeds
300 g lamb's lettuce
1 teaspoon sesame oil
200 g white mushrooms
1 apple
1 avocado
300 g cherry tomatoes
For the dressing:
salt and pepper
1/2 bunch of parsley
4 tbsp olive oil
Juice of half a lemon
1 tbsp agave syrup
2 tbsp apple juice

PREPARATION:

Wash the lamb's lettuce and spin dry. Slice the mushrooms and pit the avocado. Then peel the avocado and cut into strips. Wash the apple and remove the core. Then dice the apple. Finely chop the parsley and mix with the remaining ingredients for the dressing. Heat oil in a pan and briefly toast the sunflower seeds. Mix the lamb's lettuce, mushrooms, tomatoes and apple with the dressing. Scatter the sunflower seeds on top.

FRUITY SALAD: INGREDIENTS FOR 2 SERVINGS:

Lemon juice
100 g celery
salt and pepper
100 g apples
100 g pineapple
2 tbsp lupine yogurt
20 g of lettuce
6 walnuts

PREPARATION:

First peel the celery and cut into strips. Drizzle them with a little lemon juice. Peel the apple and remove the core. Then grate the apple and drizzle with a little lemon juice. Season the yogurt with salt and pepper. Then fold in the apples along with the celery. Then chop the walnuts and dice the pineapple. Mix both with the salad and serve the whole thing on 2 large lettuce leaves.

PASTA SALAD: INGREDIENTS FOR 2 SERVINGS:

salt and pepper
50 g whole wheat pasta
Herbs
50 g carrots

vinegar
1/2 red pepper
1 medium-sized pickle
6 black olives
1 teaspoon olive oil
2 tbsp lupine yogurt

PREPARATION:

Cook the pasta according to the instructions on the packet and rinse in cold water. Then cut the carrots, peppers and cucumber into cubes. Halve the olives. Make a marinade from the yoghurt, vinegar, olive oil, salt and pepper and let the olives steep in it. Then mix everything together and garnish with the herbs.

SPRING SALAD: INGREDIENTS FOR 2 SERVINGS:

salt and pepper
1 tbsp oregano
2 medium-sized tomatoes
1 tbsp lemon juice
1 bell pepper
1 tbsp balsamic vinegar
1/2 cucumber
1 tbsp olive oil
1 red onion
8 olives
1 chilli pepper

PREPARATION:

Wash and chop the vegetables. Cut the onion into rings. Mix everything together. Make a dressing from the olive oil, vinegar and lemon juice and add the oregano to taste. Pour the dressing over the salad and stir everything well. Finally, season the whole thing again with salt and pepper.

LENTIL CHILLI: INGREDIENTS FOR 4 SERVINGS:

Mexican spice mix as required
2 cups of red lentils
2 cans of chopped tomatoes
Vegetable broth as needed
some oil
1 can of corn
2 tbsp almond butter
3 red peppers
Chili powder
Green beans as needed
Paprika powder
1 onion
Cayenne pepper
2 cloves of garlic
pepper

PREPARATION:

Bring 4 cups of vegetable stock to the boil and let the lentils boil in it for about 10 minutes. In the meantime, fry the whole onion in a saucepan. Cut the peppers into cubes and add to the onion together with the beans. Deglaze the whole thing with the tomatoes and season. Press the garlic and add it too. Then add the corn and finally the cooked lentils. Finally stir in the almond butter and season to taste again.

CARROT AND ALMOND SOUP: INGREDIENTS FOR 2 SERVINGS:

1 heaped teaspoon dried coriander
some oil
1 pinch of salt
1 onion
1 level teaspoon instant vegetable stock
400 g carrots
1 cm of fresh ginger

100 ml almond milk

PREPARATION:

Dice the onion and ginger. Also cut the carrots into cubes. Heat the oil in a pan. Sweat the onion in it. Then add the ginger and fry together with the carrots with the lid closed for a few minutes. Dissolve the vegetable stock in the almond milk and use it to deglaze the carrots. Mix everything together well. Cook the carrots al dente over a low heat. Finally, season everything with the coriander and arrange on a plate.

POTATO SALAD WITH LEMON DRESSING: INGREDIENTS FOR 1 SERVING:

Herbs to taste
400 g waxy potatoes
1 teaspoon of hemp seeds
salt and pepper
1/2 onion
1 tsp grained vegetable broth
2 tbsp olive oil
1/2 lemon

PREPARATION:

Boil the potatoes in their skins and let them cool. Then peel and cut into slices. Mix the vegetable stock in hot water and pour over the potatoes. Squeeze the lemon and mix the lemon juice with the oil and spices. Cut the onion into rings and add to the potatoes together with the hemp seeds. Then spread the dressing over it and mix everything well.

FRIED BROCCOLI: INGREDIENTS FOR 2 SERVINGS:

Salt and cayenne pepper
some rapeseed oil
1 tsp grained vegetable broth

1 red onion
2 heaped teaspoons of chestnut flour
500 g broccoli
150 ml almond milk
400 g mushrooms

PREPARATION:

Separate the florets from the broccoli. Cut the mushrooms into slices and dice the onion. Cook the broccoli, heat the oil in a pan and fry the onion in it. Then add the mushrooms and fry. Season everything with the vegetable stock, salt and cayenne pepper. Deglaze the mushrooms with half of the almond milk and add the finished broccoli. Mix everything well. Mix the chestnut flour with the remaining almond milk until smooth and stir into the vegetables.

BELL PEPPER PAN: INGREDIENTS FOR 1 SERVING:

1 cm ginger
150 g red pointed peppers
1 pinch of salt
150 g green pointed peppers
1 teaspoon coconut flour
150 g white pointed peppers
100 ml creamy coconut milk
1 teaspoon coconut oil
1 clove of garlic
1 onion

PREPARATION:

Wash and core the peppers. Cut the pulp into strips. Halve the onion and also cut into slices. Cut the garlic and ginger into fine cubes. Heat the coconut oil in a pan and steam the onion. Then add the ginger and garlic. Then add the peppers and heat everything for a few minutes while stirring. Deglaze with the coconut milk and reduce the heat. Let cook with the lid closed. Finally, season everything with salt.

POTATO AND VEGETABLE STEW: INGREDIENTS FOR 2 SERVINGS:

2 tsp sambal oelek
some oil
200 ml vegetable broth
1 onion
300 ml almond milk
6 small potatoes
2 large, red pointed peppers
500 g broccoli

PREPARATION:

Divide the broccoli into florets. Peel the potatoes and the onion and cut into cubes. Core and dice the peppers. Heat some oil in a saucepan. Steam the onion in it. Then add the potatoes and fry them. Then add the remaining vegetables. Deglaze everything with the almond milk and vegetable stock. Finally, season the stew with the sambal oelek. Cook the whole thing with the lid closed and low heat until the desired consistency is achieved.

BROCCOLI AND ALMOND PAN: INGREDIENTS FOR 2 SERVINGS:

1 pinch of salt
500 g broccoli
1 handful of sliced almonds
100 ml almond milk

Preparation:

First cut the broccoli into florets. Cover the bottom of a pan with almond milk. Then add the broccoli and almonds. Bring everything to the boil and cook over a low heat until the broccoli is tender. Finally, season the whole thing with salt.

CARROT AND PEPPER PAN WITH COCONUT SAUCE: INGREDIENTS FOR 1 SERVING:

1 pinch of salt
1 tbsp oil
4 teaspoons coriander
1 onion
2 tbsp creamy coconut milk
250 g carrots
1 tbsp lemon juice
150 g light green peppers

PREPARATION:

Peel and dice the onion and carrots. Wash the peppers and remove the seeds. Also cut the pulp into cubes. Heat the oil in a pan. Sauté the onion until translucent. Then add the carrots and put the lid on the pan. As soon as the carrots are al dente, add the peppers to the pan and close the lid again. In the meantime, stir the coconut milk with the lemon juice. Add the lemon and coconut milk mixture to the vegetables and stir. Cook everything with the lid closed until the desired firmness is achieved. Season with the coriander and salt.

BELL PEPPER AND CHICKPEA SALAD: INGREDIENTS FOR 1 SERVING:

1 pinch of rose-hot paprika powder
1 can of chickpeas
1/4 teaspoon garam masala
1 tbsp lemon juice
1/4 teaspoon cumin
1 tbsp neutral oil
1/4 teaspoon salt
1 spring onion
1 pinch of chili powder
1/4 teaspoon turmeric
1 bell pepper

PREPARATION:

First wash and chop the peppers. Clean the spring onions and cut into thin rings. Mix the chickpeas and the juice together with the oil, lemon juice, spring onions and bell pepper. Season the whole thing with the spices. Let the salad steep before serving.

MILK SOUP WITH CORIANDER: INGREDIENTS FOR 1 SERVING:

salt
4 coriander leaves
1 tsp grained vegetable broth
300 ml of plant milk
1 tbsp oil

Preparation:

Wash the coriander leaves well. Heat the oil in a pan. Put on the coriander leaves in it. Deglaze everything with the milk. Season to taste with the vegetable stock and salt and simmer everything over low heat with the lid closed. Always stir. Finally puree the whole thing.

GLASS NOODLES WITH VEGETABLES: INGREDIENTS FOR 2 SERVINGS:

1 handful of cashew nuts
1 onion
1 tbsp coconut oil
1 leek
2 tbsp sweet soy sauce
2 carrots
2 tbsp tamari sauce
1 handful of broccoli florets
50 g glass noodles

PREPARATION:

Cut the onion into small pieces. Heat oil in a pan. Sauté the onions in it. In the meantime, cut the carrots and leek into strips. Soak the glass noodles in hot water. Add the carrots to the onions and sauté. Then add the leek, the tamari sauce and the soy sauce. Then put the broccoli in the pan and cook everything with the lid closed. Cut the glass noodles in the water, drain and add to the vegetables. Mix everything together well.

SIMPLE FRIED POTATOES: INGREDIENTS FOR 2 SERVINGS:

salt
1 leek
350 g potatoes
1 red onion
3 tbsp oil

Preparation:

Peel and dice the potatoes. Split and wash the leek. Then cut the leek into short strips. Chop the onion into small pieces. Heat the oil in a pan. Steam the onions in it. Then add the potatoes and fry while turning. Then add the leek and fry as well. Finally, season the fried potatoes with salt.

SPICY VEGETABLE POT: INGREDIENTS FOR 1 SERVING:

50 ml creamy coconut milk
1 tbsp oil
1 level teaspoon of green curry paste
230 g white radish
230 g carrots

PREPARATION:

Cut the radish and carrots into thin strips. Heat oil in a saucepan. Toast the curry paste in it. Then add the vegetables and fry, turning constantly. Then turn down the heat and seal the pot. Steam the vegetables. Gradually stir in the coconut milk. Bring everything to the boil and serve.

BAKED ZUCCHINI PAN: INGREDIENTS FOR 1 SERVING:

2 tbsp fried onions
2 tbsp liquid coconut oil
50 g cheese substitute
1 zucchini
3 tbsp oat cream
200 g fresh, brown mushrooms
salt and pepper
some leek

PREPARATION:

First wash the zucchini and cut into slices together with the mushrooms. Cut the leek into rings. Heat the coconut oil in a pan. Fry the zucchini in it. Then add the mushrooms and fry them too. Then add the leek and steam. Deglaze the whole thing with the oat cream and stir. Season everything to taste with the spices. Then fold in the cheese. Finally, distribute the fried onions on top and mix everything together.

VEGETABLE ROULADES: INGREDIENTS FOR 2 SERVINGS:

salt and pepper
400 g potatoes
1 pinch of nutmeg
200 g pumpkin
1 pinch of cayenne pepper
1 red pepper
3 tbsp oil
1 zucchini
200 ml vegetable broth
2 cloves of garlic
200 ml vegetable broth
1 can of chunky tomatoes
5 large savoy cabbage leaves

1 onion

PREPARATION:

Let the savoy cabbage leaves cook in boiling salted water for about 4-5 minutes. Then rinse with cold water and roll dry with a rolling pin. Peel and dice the potatoes. Then boil them in salted water and then pour them off. Mash the potatoes and season with nutmeg. Prepare the pumpkin according to the same principle. Then season the pumpkin with cayenne pepper. Dice the onion and sauté in a saucepan with oil. Deglaze these with the tomatoes and add the stock. Let the whole thing boil for a few minutes and then put in a baking dish. Fry the garlic with a little oil and add the peppers. Season everything with salt and pepper. Stuff the savoy cabbage leaves with the potato mixture, pumpkin mixture and diced paprika and roll up. Then place the finished roulades in the baking dish with the open end facing down. Finally, brush everything with a little oil and bake for about 40 minutes at 180-200 ° C.

COLORFUL, HEALTHY PAN: INGREDIENTS FOR 2 SERVINGS:

1 heaped tablespoon of granulated broth
some oil
200 g broccoli
1 onion
220 g potatoes
3 cm ginger
220 g carrots

PREPARATION:

Divide the broccoli into florets. Cut the ginger into sticks and cut the potatoes and carrots into "French fries". Chop the onion into small pieces. Heat the oil in a pan. Steam the onion in it. Then add the ginger and fry. Then add the potatoes and cook everything over medium heat with the lid closed for about 5 minutes. Then add the broccoli florets and stir everything well. Season the whole thing and close the lid again and steam until the vegetables have the desired firmness.

LIGHT POINTED PEPPER SOUP: INGREDIENTS FOR 3 SERVINGS:

500 ml vegetable broth
some oil
1 red onion
4 red pointed peppers

Preparation:

Wash the peppers and remove the seeds. Cut the pulp into small pieces. Cut the onion into small cubes. Heat the oil in a saucepan. Sauté the onions in it. Then add the peppers and let them sweat. Always stir. Deglaze the whole thing with the vegetable stock and let it simmer. Puree everything at the end.

FRIED POTATOES WITH KOHLRABI: INGREDIENTS FOR 2 SERVINGS:

salt and pepper
500 g kohlrabi
some oil
200 g potatoes
100 ml almond milk
2 heaped teaspoons of wild garlic paste

PREPARATION:

Peel and cut the kohlrabi and potatoes. Heat oil in a pan. Fry the kohlrabi in it. Then add the potatoes and fry them. Mix the wild garlic paste with the almond milk and add to the vegetables. Let everything simmer with the lid closed and low heat. Finally, season the whole thing with salt and pepper.

POTATO AND CELERY STEW: INGREDIENTS FOR 4 SERVINGS:

salt and pepper
20 g green spelled
nutmeg
2 onions
Cayenne pepper
4 carrots
lukewarm water
1.5 kg predominantly waxy potatoes
1/2 celeriac
3 thyme stalks
4 bunches of parsley
2 tbsp vegetable oil
4 tbsp vegetable stock powder

PREPARATION:

Peel and dice the onions, carrots, celery and potatoes. Heat oil in a
saucepan. Fry the vegetables together with the green spelled. Then add
the thyme with a spice bag to the pot. Deglaze with the stock and
water. Let it cook until the potatoes are soft. Then remove the
thyme. Chop the parsley and season the stew with the remaining herbs.

PUMPKIN SOUP: INGREDIENTS FOR 4 SERVINGS:

salt and pepper
1 heaped tbsp coconut oil
1 heaped teaspoon red curry paste
1 hokkaido pumpkin
200 ml almond milk
3 red peppers
400 ml vegetable broth

PREPARATION:

Wash and core the peppers. Cut the pulp into cubes. Wash the pumpkin too and remove the seeds. Then dice the pumpkin. Heat the coconut oil in a saucepan. Sweat the pumpkin in it. Then add the paprika and deglaze the whole thing with the vegetable stock. Bring everything to the boil and continue to simmer. In the meantime, mix the almond milk with the curry paste. Add the mixture to the soup and cook until the vegetables are soft. Then puree everything and season with salt and pepper.

RAW VEGETABLES WITH BROWN MILLET: INGREDIENTS FOR 2 SERVINGS:

1 pinch of chili powder
250 ml vegan yogurt
12 peppermint leaves
6 heaped teaspoons of ground brown millet
1 tbsp lemon juice
1 carrot
8 dried figs
4 parsnips

PREPARATION:

Mix the brown millet with the yogurt. Peel the carrots, figs and parsnips and cut into sticks. Add both to the yogurt mixture. Chop the peppermint leaves very finely and add them to the vegetables together with the lemon juice. Mix everything together well and season with the chili powder.

DILL SOUP: INGREDIENTS FOR 2 SERVINGS:

Lemon juice
oil
1 bunch of dill
1 onion
3 heaped teaspoons of grained vegetable stock

500 ml of vegetable milk

PREPARATION:

Heat the oil in a pot. Finely dice the onion and sauté in the oil. Mix the milk with the vegetable stock. Wash and finely chop the dill. Deglaze the onion with the milk and add the dill. Mix everything well and bring to the boil briefly. Finally, season the soup with lemon juice.

BEETROOT ON SPINACH: INGREDIENTS FOR 1 SERVING:

1 handful of herbs
200 g pre-cooked beetroot
1 tbsp oil
50 g fresh baby spinach
salt and pepper
1 handful of walnuts
1 shot of crema di balsamic vinegar
1 red onion

PREPARATION:

First cut the beetroot into small pieces. Mix the walnuts with the beetroot juice and the finely chopped beetroot. Preheat the oven to 170 ° C. Cut the onion into thin slices. Grease a baking dish with oil and spread the onion in it. Put the whole thing in the oven for about 10 minutes. In the meantime, wash the spinach and place on a plate. Season with salt and pepper. Put the finished onions on a plate and pour the beetroot-walnut mixture into the baking dish. Drizzle with the crema di balsamic vinegar and sprinkle the onions over the top. Put everything back in the oven for about 20 minutes. Finally, spread the beetroot over the spinach.

MUSHROOM PAN: INGREDIENTS FOR 2 SERVINGS:

4 heaping tablespoons of horseradish

2 tbsp ghee
250 g mushrooms
1 onion
2 potatoes
2 cloves of garlic
350 g carrots

PREPARATION:

Heat the ghee in a pan. Chop the onion and garlic into small pieces. Sauté both in the pan until translucent. Cut the carrots into sticks and dice the potatoes. Wash and slice the mushrooms. Add the carrots to the onions and fry for a few minutes with the lid closed. Then add the potatoes and close the pan again. Then add the mushrooms and fry everything again with the lid closed. Then reduce the heat and steam the vegetables. Finally add the horseradish and stir everything well. Season everything with salt and pepper before serving.

CELERY AND PEPPER PAN: INGREDIENTS FOR 1 SERVING:

1 heaped teaspoon of granulated broth
1 tbsp coconut oil
100 ml of water
300 g celery
1/2 pk. Herbal mixture
2 red pointed peppers

PREPARATION:

Cut the celery into cubes. Core the peppers and also cut into cubes. Heat the oil in a pan. Fry the celery in it. Then add the bell pepper and pour the vegetable stock over it. Let the whole thing fry briefly with the lid closed. Then deglaze with water and let everything cook. Finally season with the herbs and stir.

VEGETABLE PATTIES: INGREDIENTS FOR 2 SERVINGS:

oil
300 g Hokkaido pumpkin
pepper
300 g carrots
2 teaspoons of curry powder
200 g peppers
3 tsp vegetable broth
1 onion
6 teaspoons of flour
2 cloves of garlic

PREPARATION:

Finely grate the pumpkin and carrots. Finely chop the peppers, onions and garlic. Mix all ingredients together. Shape the mixture into small balls and flatten them a little. Fry the patties in a pan with fat.

PUMPKIN STEW: INGREDIENTS FOR 2 SERVINGS:

2 teaspoons ground tiger nuts
oil
200 ml vegetable broth
2 leeks
1/2 hokkaido pumpkin

Preparation:

Cut the leek into rings. Core and dice the pumpkin. Heat the oil in a pot. Fry the leek. Then add the pumpkin and stir everything together. Deglaze with the vegetable stock and let cook. Stir in the tiger nuts before serving.

POTATO SOUP: INGREDIENTS FOR 2 SERVINGS:

1 pinch of nutmeg

2 kohlrabi

oil

2 onions

500 ml vegetable broth

300 g potatoes

Preparation:

Wash the stems and the green leaves of the kohlrabi and cut into small pieces. Heat the oil in a pot. Finely dice the onion and sauté in it. Then add the kohlrabi leaves and stems and fry. Deglaze the whole thing with the vegetable stock. Peel and chop the potatoes. Put these in the pot and bring to the boil briefly. Let everything simmer at a low temperature. As soon as the vegetables are soft, puree the whole thing and season with nutmeg.

CUCUMBER SALAD: INGREDIENTS FOR 1 SERVING:

1/4 cucumber

chives

1 tomato

basil

1/2 green pepper

1 bunch of spring onions

For the marinade:

2-3 tbsp olive oil

1 tbsp wine vinegar

salt and pepper

PREPARATION:

Wash the cucumber and cut into sticks. Cut the tomato into wedges. Core the peppers and cut into sticks. Cut the onions into rings and finely chop the basil and chives. Mix everything together. Mix all ingredients for the marinade and pour over the salad.

POTATO SALAD: INGREDIENTS FOR 4 SERVINGS:

chives
750 g of fat potatoes
1 teaspoon mustard
2 tbsp cider vinegar
salt and pepper
3 tbsp sunflower oil
100 g onions
5 tbsp beef soup

PREPARATION:

Wash the potatoes and put them in cold water with salt. Boil the potatoes in it until soft, then rinse and peel. Cut the potatoes into slices. Chop the onions and mix with the rest of the ingredients. Mix everything with the still warm potatoes and garnish with chives before serving.

SPRING ROLLS: INGREDIENTS FOR 4 PERSONS:

salt and pepper
1 packet of rice paper for spring rolls
olive oil
3 carrots
Chilli flakes
1 cucumber
1 packet of cress
1 package of green asparagus
1 red pepper
For the dip:
3 teaspoons of pink berries
1 pk. Herbal Hollandaise

PREPARATION:

Wash and core the peppers. Cut the pulp into strips. Heat the oil in a pan. Wash the asparagus and cut off the ends. Cook the asparagus in the pan for about 4–6 minutes. Then quench in ice water. Peel the carrots and cut into sticks. Peel the cucumber and remove the seeds. Cut these into strips as well. Mix everything together and serve.

BEETROOT SALAD: INGREDIENTS FOR 2 SERVINGS:

salt and pepper
2 cooked beetroot
Lemon juice
1 lettuce heart
2 stalks of spring onions
4 red tomatoes
1 tbsp chopped parsley
4 yellow tomatoes
1 tbsp nut oil
3 tbsp pomegranate seeds
2 tsp hot mustard
2 tbsp cashew nuts
2 tbsp pomegranate syrup

PREPARATION:

Mix the pomegranate syrup, mustard and oil. Season the vinaigrette with salt, pepper and a little lemon juice. Roughly chop the cashew nuts and toast them in a pan without fat. Wash and dry the lettuce heart. Remove the yellow leaves from the stalk. Wash the tomatoes and spring onions and then cut them into slices. Wash and finely chop the parsley. Cut one of the beetroot into slices and arrange on a plate. Dice the rest of the beetroot and place in the center of the plate. Drape the lettuce heart and tomatoes around. Sprinkle the whole thing with the dressing. Finally sprinkle the parsley, spring onions and cashew nuts on top.

GRAPEFRUIT SALAD: INGREDIENTS FOR 4 PERSONS:

Chilli flakes
1 teaspoon aniseed
salt and pepper
3 red onions
50 ml grapefruit juice
1 bunch of spring onions
10 tbsp olive oil
2 bulbs of fennel with green
1 lime
2 rosé grapefruit

PREPARATION:

For the marinade, roast the anise seeds in a pan without fat. Chop the fennel greens. Fillet the grapefruit while collecting the juice. Squeeze the lime. Mix the olive oil with the grapefruit juice, the lime juice, the fennel green and the aniseed. Season to taste with salt, pepper and chilli flakes. Wash the fennel, remove the inner stalk and slice the fennel into strips. Peel and finely slice the onions. Mix the onions and fennel with the marinade. Wash the spring onions and cut into thin rings. Use the green as well. Arrange the salad and spread the grapefruit wedges over it. Sprinkle the whole thing with the spring onions and let sit in the fridge for 15 minutes.

SPINACH SOUP: INGREDIENTS FOR 2 SERVINGS:

fresh coriander
500 g fresh spinach
peanuts
1 can of coconut milk
salt and pepper
1 onion
Chili powder
1 tbsp peanut butter

some ginger
2 tbsp lemon juice
2 tbsp vegetable stock powder
200 ml almond milk

PREPARATION:

Cut the onion and ginger into small pieces. Fry both in a little coconut oil. Wash the spinach and add it together with the coconut milk, almond milk and vegetable stock powder. Let the whole thing simmer for about 10 minutes. Finally puree everything and season with the lemon juice, salt, pepper, peanut butter and the chili powder. Chop the peanuts and garnish the soup with the peanuts and coriander.

FRIES WITH MAYONNAISE WITH A DIFFERENCE: INGREDIENTS FOR 2 SERVINGS:

salt and pepper
2 celery bulbs
1 teaspoon vegetable stock powder
2 tbsp coconut oil
2 tbsp lemon juice
1 soft avocado
approx. 50 ml almond milk

PREPARATION:

Peel the celery and cut into sticks. Heat the coconut oil in a pan. Fry the celery in it for about 20 minutes. In the meantime, peel and stone the avocado. Puree the pulp with the lemon juice and almond milk. Season the whole thing with the spices and the vegetable stock powder.

CARROT PUDDING: INGREDIENTS FOR 4 SERVINGS:

Pistachios
300 g carrots

2 tbsp rose water
400 ml almond milk
6–8 dates
1 teaspoon Indian spice mix "Garam Masala"
3 tbsp corn starch
1 teaspoon vanilla powder

PREPARATION:

First peel the carrots and cut them into small pieces. Puree 200 ml almond milk with the dates and carrots. Bring the whole thing to the boil in a saucepan with the remaining almond milk, corn starch, spice mixture and vanilla. Season the pudding with the rose water and sprinkle the pistachios over it.

VEGETABLE SPAGHETTI WITH MUSHROOM SAUCE: INGREDIENTS FOR 2 PEOPLE:

salt and pepper
2 sweet potatoes
Chili powder
300 g mushrooms
1 tbsp vegetable stock powder
400 ml almond milk
2 tbsp yeast flakes
1 tbsp coconut oil
2 tbsp almond butter
1 tbsp coconut oil
1 onion

PREPARATION:

Preheat the oven to 170 ° C. Peel the potatoes and use the spiral cutter to make spaghetti. Place these on a baking sheet lined with baking paper and bake the spaghetti for about 25 minutes. In the meantime, cut the onion into small pieces. Heat the coconut oil in a pan and fry the onion in it. Then add the mushrooms, almond milk, almond butter, spices and vegetable stock. Puree the whole thing and heat it over low heat. Finally stir in the yeast flakes.

Potato and pointed cabbage pan with coconut milk

INGREDIENTS FOR 2 SERVINGS:: SALT AND PEPPER

6 potatoes
1 pointed cabbage
150 ml coconut milk
1 bell pepper
1 tsp curry
2 carrots
2 teaspoons of turmeric
2 onions
2 tbsp olive oil

PREPARATION:

Wash the cabbage and remove the stalk. Then cut the cabbage into fine strips. Peel and dice the onions. Peel and dice the potatoes and carrots. Wash the peppers and cut into strips. Heat the oil in a pan. Fry the onions in it. Then add the carrots and potatoes. Fry everything for about 10 minutes. Then add the cabbage and cook for another 3 minutes. Cook the cabbage over low heat. Finally stir in the coconut milk and bring to the boil. Season to taste with the spices and serve.

QUINOA WITH PEANUT SAUCE: INGREDIENTS FOR 2 SERVINGS:

30 g pomegranate seeds
100 g quinoa
50 g baby spinach
1 tsp turmeric powder
1 tbsp peanut kernels
salt and pepper
1 pinch of chilli flakes
1/2 celeriac

1 tbsp peanut butter
1 carrot
100 g lupine yogurt
1 teaspoon olive oil
2 parsley stalks
dried thyme
Paprika powder
dried marjoram

PREPARATION:

Rinse the quinoa and cook for 15 minutes with twice the amount of salted water and turmeric. Then let the quinoa soak. In the meantime, peel and dice the celery and carrots. Heat the oil in a pan. Steam the vegetables in it for about 10 minutes over medium heat. Season the vegetables with the spices, salt and pepper. Wash the parsley and shake dry. Then finely chop the parsley. Mix the peanut butter with the yogurt and half of the parsley. Season the whole thing with salt, pepper and the chilli flakes. Chop the peanuts. Serve the spinach with the quinoa. Spread the vegetables on top and drizzle with the sauce. Garnish with the rest of the parsley, the peanuts and the pomegranate seeds.

VEGETABLE SOUP WITH POTATOES: INGREDIENTS FOR 2 SERVINGS:

1 pinch of cayenne pepper
250 g celery
125 ml coconut milk
200 g potatoes
1/2 teaspoon turmeric powder
1 onion
salt and pepper
1 piece of ginger
2 carrots
2 tbsp coconut oil
500 ml vegetable broth

PREPARATION:

Wash, peel and chop the vegetables, except for the carrots, and the ginger. Approx. Dice 50 g celery. Heat oil in a saucepan. Steam the onion and then the ginger in it. Then add the vegetables and steam them too. Deglaze with the broth and cook over medium heat for about 15 minutes. In the meantime, peel and dice the carrots. Heat 1 tablespoon of oil in a pan. Fry the carrots and the celery cubes for 7 minutes. Season everything with turmeric, salt and pepper. Add the coconut milk to the soup and puree the soup. Season everything with salt, pepper and cayenne pepper. Finally add the diced vegetables and stir.

POTATO AND BRUSSELS SPROUTS PANCAKES: INGREDIENTS FOR 2–3 PEOPLE:

Rock salt
1 kg of Brussels sprouts
600 g potatoes
nutmeg
1 tbsp grated almonds
mace
1 tbsp coconut oil
black pepper
Juice of half a lemon
Smoked salt

PREPARATION:

Clean the Brussels sprouts. Melt the coconut oil in a saucepan. Roast the Brussels sprouts in it with the lid closed. Then add the lemon juice. Deglaze the Brussels sprouts with the smoked salt and 100 ml of water. Cook the Brussels sprouts for about 15 minutes, stirring gently. Then season with pepper, nutmeg and mace to taste. Peel and grate the potatoes. Fold the almonds and salt into the potato mixture. Heat the oil in a pan. Press the potato mixture into the pan. Spread the Brussels sprouts on top and press in gently. Cover the pan with a lid and fry the potato and Brussels sprouts fritters over medium heat. Then turn the pancake and fry from the other side. Finally sprinkle with parsley and serve.

OVEN BAKED VEGETABLES: INGREDIENTS FOR 2 SERVINGS:

some parsley leaves
450 g carrots
1 tbsp sunflower seeds
320 g fennel
2 tbsp olive oil
300 g red onions
1/2 teaspoon pepper
1/2 teaspoon hot paprika powder
1 teaspoon salt
1 tbsp lemon juice
1 tbsp agave syrup
2 tbsp balsamic vinegar

PREPARATION:

First preheat the oven to 220 ° C. Peel the carrots and cut in half lengthways. Peel the onions. Wash the fennel and remove the stem. Then cut the onions and fennel into wedges. Mix the vegetables with 2 tablespoons of olive oil and salt. Spread the vegetables on a baking sheet and cook in the oven for about 30–40 minutes. In the meantime, mix the agave syrup with the lemon juice, balsamic vinegar, pepper and paprika powder. Spread the dressing over the finished vegetables and serve. Sprinkle with the parsley and sunflower seeds.

CHICKPEA AND ZUCCHINI PAN: INGREDIENTS FOR 2 SERVINGS:

salt and pepper
3 zucchini
1 teaspoon of yeast flakes
1 can of chickpeas
1 pinch of cayenne pepper

1 clove of garlic
1-2 tablespoons chopped parsley
1 tbsp olive oil
1-2 tbsp sesame seeds

PREPARATION:

Cut the zucchini into slices. Heat the oil in a pan. Fry the zucchini in it for about 5 minutes. Allow the chickpeas to drain off. Peel the garlic and cut into cubes. Add the garlic with the chickpeas to the zucchini and sauté for another 5 minutes. Finally, season everything with the herbs, sesame seeds and spices.

EGGPLANT CHICKPEAS OUT OF THE OVEN: INGREDIENTS FOR 2 SERVINGS:

2 tbsp pistachios
400 g eggplant
2 tbsp pomegranate
100 g pre-cooked chickpeas
1/4 teaspoon smoked paprika powder
1 red onion
1/4 teaspoon pepper
1 clove of garlic
1/2 teaspoon salt
50 g Swiss chard
1 tbsp lemon juice
1 tsp sambal oelek
1 tbsp agave syrup
1 teaspoon sesame oil
2 tbsp olive oil
For the dressing:
1/4 teaspoon salt
1 tbsp lemon juice
1 tbsp water
1 teaspoon tahini
2 tbsp lupine yogurt

PREPARATION:

First preheat the oven to 180 ° C. In the meantime, cut the eggplant into cubes and the onion into rings. Chop the garlic. Mix the aubergine with the sambal oelek, the olive oil, the lemon juice, the sesame oil, the agave syrup, salt and pepper as well as the paprika powder. Then mix in the onions, garlic and chickpeas. Spread the vegetables on a baking sheet and bake for 20 minutes. Mix all ingredients for the dressing together. Wash the chard and arrange on plates. Spread the vegetables on top and pour the dressing on top. Finally, garnish with the pistachios and pomegranate.

HERBAL POLENTA WITH ASPARAGUS: INGREDIENTS FOR 2 SERVINGS:

Pine nuts
500 g green asparagus
2 tbsp lemon juice
4–6 sage leaves
1 onion
5 stalks of lemon thyme
1 garlic yeast
1 tbsp vegetable margarine
120 g minute polenta
1/2 teaspoon freshly ground nutmeg
500 ml of water
1 tbsp yeast flakes
1/2 teaspoon salt
1 pinch of pepper

PREPARATION:

First wash the asparagus. Cut off the dry ends. Place the asparagus on a baking sheet and season with salt, pepper and lemon juice. Spread 1 tablespoon of oil over it. Bake the asparagus for 12–15 minutes at 180 ° C. In the meantime, finely chop the onion and garlic. Heat 1 tablespoon of oil in a saucepan. Steam the onion and garlic in it. Deglaze everything with water and stir in the polenta. Season everything with nutmeg, yeast flakes, salt and pepper. Let the polenta simmer for 5 minutes. Pluck the thyme from the stalks and cut the sage. Stir the margarine and herbs into the polenta. Mix everything well and let it steep. Arrange the polenta and serve the asparagus on top. Put the pine nuts and a little lemon juice on top.

GRAPE AND VEGETABLE SALAD: INGREDIENTS FOR 2 SERVINGS:

2 tbsp nuts
2 carrots
150 g of grapes
250 g beetroot
60 g spinach
For the vinaigrette:
salt and pepper
2 tbsp lemon juice
6 mint leaves
2 tbsp olive oil
1 teaspoon mustard
1 tbsp agave syrup

PREPARATION:

Peel the carrots and beetroot and cut into strips. Halve the grapes. Mix the beetroot, carrots and grapes with the nuts. Chop the mint and mix with the remaining ingredients for the vinaigrette. Pour the vinaigrette over the salad and sprinkle some nuts over it.

GREEN BOWL WITH FRIED POTATOES: INGREDIENTS FOR 2 SERVINGS:

salt and pepper
500 g small, boiled potatoes
Paprika powder
200 g baby broccoli
Cayenne pepper
1 romaine lettuce

3 tbsp frying oil
1 clove of garlic
1/2 avocado
<u>For the dressing:</u>
cress
40 g cashew nuts
some lemon juice
80 ml of water
salt and pepper
1 1/2 tsp miso paste
Juice of half a lemon
3 tbsp olive oil

PREPARATION:

Soak the cashew nuts for 2 hours. Wash the broccoli. Heat 1 tablespoon of oil in a pan. Cook the broccoli in it for 10–12 minutes until al dente. Cut the garlic and add to the broccoli for the last 5 minutes. Season with salt and pepper. Halve the potatoes and fry in a pan with 1 tablespoon of oil for 10 minutes. Season the potatoes with salt and pepper as well as with paprika powder and a little cayenne pepper. Remove the stalk from the romaine lettuce. Halve the salad and fry for 3–5 minutes. Drain the cashew nuts. Mix and puree all ingredients for the dressing. Pit the avocado and cut into slices. Mix everything and serve.

SAVOY-CURRY PAN WITH COCONUT MILK: INGREDIENTS FOR 2 SERVINGS:

salt and pepper
250 g savoy cabbage
1 tsp green curry paste
1 small zucchini
150 ml creamy coconut milk

PREPARATION:

Clean the savoy cabbage and cut into thin strips. Finely chop the zucchini. Mix the coconut milk with the curry paste in a saucepan and heat. Cook the savoy cabbage and zucchini over medium heat with the lid closed. Finally, season everything with salt and pepper.

WARM SALAD: INGREDIENTS FOR 2 SERVINGS:

salt and pepper
1 kohlrabi
parsley
2 potatoes
olive oil

Preparation:

Clean and dice the kohlrabi. Cook the kohlrabi cubes in a little salted water. In the meantime, peel the potatoes, dice them and cook them. Mix the finished kohlrabi and the finished potatoes. Spread some olive oil over it. Finely chop the parsley and season the warm salad with salt, pepper and parsley.

VEGETABLE JELLIES: INGREDIENTS FOR 4 PERSONS:

1 pinch of herbal salt
2 carrots
1 pinch of black clover
2 spring onions
1 pinch of marjoram
1 clove of garlic
1 tsp agar agar
1/2 red pepper
1 tbsp fresh, chopped herbs
1/2 yellow pepper
500 ml vegetable broth without yeast
2 tbsp peas

PREPARATION:

Cut the carrots into sticks. Slice the spring onions, dice the peppers and press the garlic. Cook all the vegetables except the peas in the vegetable stock. Then stir in agar-agar. Let everything cook for 2 minutes. Then add the peas, spices and herbs. Then fill everything into molds and let the brawn cool.

BAKED CARROTS AND PARSNIPS: INGREDIENTS FOR 4 SERVINGS:

3 sprigs of rosemary
500 g parsnips
Seasoned Salt
300 g carrots
5 tbsp coconut oil
Preparation:
First preheat the oven to 200 ° C. Cut the carrots and parsnips into sticks. Spread both on a baking sheet and season with salt. Halve the rosemary sprigs and distribute between the vegetables. Drizzle everything with a little coconut oil and cook in the oven for 30 minutes.

MANGO SALAD: INGREDIENTS:

Juice of half a lemon
2 mangoes
200 g papaya
Preparation:
Peel the fruit and remove the stones. Dice the pulp. Halve the lemon and squeeze it. Drizzle the fruit cubes with the lemon juice. Mix everything together and let it steep for about half an hour.

COOKED POTATOES: INGREDIENTS FOR 2 SERVINGS:

salt and pepper
550 g potatoes
1 teaspoon marjoram
300 ml vegetable broth
1 pinch of chilli flakes
2 tbsp coconut oil

1 teaspoon paprika powder, noble sweet

PREPARATION:

Peel and dice the potatoes. Heat the coconut oil in a pan. Fry the potatoes in it for 3–5 minutes and season with the spices. Then deglaze with the vegetable stock. Let everything simmer for about 15 minutes over medium heat. Stir again and again. Finally, season the potatoes again and serve.

Spaghetti with tomato sauce is a little different

INGREDIENTS FOR 2 SERVINGS:: SPICES

2 zucchini
Hemp cream
4 carrots
garlic
3 tomatoes
Vegetable oil
Onions

Preparation:

Cut the carrots into spaghetti with a spiral cutter. Boil these in a little salted water. In the meantime, dice the onions and garlic cloves. Heat the oil in a pan. Sauté the garlic and onions in it. Dice the tomatoes and add to the onions. Season everything with the spices. Deglaze the tomatoes with the cream. Drain the carrot spaghetti and mix into the sauce.

VEGETABLE STICKS: INGREDIENTS:

Vegetable oil
Parsnips
rosemary
Carrots
Onions
paprika

Preparation:

Wash the vegetables. Peel the parsnips and carrots. Core the peppers. Cut the vegetables into sticks. Dice the onions. Mix the rosemary with the vegetable oil and the onions. Then fold in the vegetables. Spread everything on a baking sheet and bake at 180 ° C until the vegetable sticks are lightly brown.

BEANS WITH SESAME SEEDS: INGREDIENTS FOR 4 SERVINGS:

salt and pepper
600 g French beans
olive oil
3 spring onions
Juice and zest of half a lemon
1/2 chilli pepper
2 tbsp sesame oil
2 tbsp sesame seeds

PREPARATION:

Chop the beans and cook in salted water for 10 minutes. Cut the spring onions into rings. Core the chilli pepper and cut into rings. Heat the sesame oil in a pan. Steam the spring onions and the chilli pepper for 5 minutes while turning. Then stir in the lemon juice and lemon zest. Add the finished beans and season everything with salt and pepper. Steam for 10 minutes. Toast the sesame seeds in a pan. Arrange the beans on a plate and sprinkle the sesame seeds on top.

BRUSSELS SPROUTS WITH ALMONDS: INGREDIENTS FOR 4 SERVINGS:

salt and pepper
700 g Brussels sprouts
2 tbsp spelled breadcrumbs
100 g of chopped almonds
50 g butter
1 clove of garlic
Zest of a lemon

PREPARATION:

First clean the Brussels sprouts and cut off the bottom. Cook the Brussels sprouts in salted water for 5–7 minutes. Then keep the cabbage warm. Heat half of the butter in a pan. Roast the almonds and halved garlic in it. Season the garlic with salt, pepper and lemon zest. Then remove the garlic and put everything aside. Heat the rest of the butter in a saucepan. Toast the breadcrumbs in it. Add the breadcrumbs to the almond mixture. Serve the Brussels sprouts and spread the almond and breadcrumb mixture over them.

POTATO AND KALE STEW: INGREDIENTS FOR 2 SERVINGS:

salt and pepper
250 g kale
ground thyme
250 g potatoes
2 tbsp coconut oil
2 tomatoes
500 ml vegetable stock (without yeast)
2 onions
2 cloves of garlic

PREPARATION:

Clean the cabbage and cut into strips. Cut the potatoes into cubes. Peel the tomatoes and dice the pulp. Finely chop the onions and garlic. Heat coconut oil in a saucepan. Steam the onions and garlic in it. Then add the potatoes and cook for 2 minutes. Deglaze everything with the vegetable stock and season with salt. Simmer for 10 minutes with the lid closed. Then add the kale and cook for 15 minutes. Then add the tomatoes and cook for 3 minutes. Finally season everything with pepper, salt and thyme.

BEAN PAN: INGREDIENTS FOR 4 SERVINGS:

salt and pepper
700 g potatoes
3 tbsp olive oil
500 g green beans
2 sprigs of savory
2 onions
2 sprigs of thyme

PREPARATION:

Wash the potatoes and cook in salted boiling water for 20 minutes. In the meantime, wash the beans and cut them into small pieces. Blanch these in boiling salted water for 8 minutes. Peel the onions and cut into rings. Wash the herbs and gently shake dry. Rinse the finished beans in cold water and let them drain. Drain the potatoes and let them cool. Then peel the potatoes and cut them into slices. Heat 2 tablespoons of oil in a pan and fry the potatoes in it. Season the potatoes with salt and pepper. Heat the remaining oil in a separate pan. Fry the beans, onions, thyme and savory for 8–10 minutes. Then fold everything under the potatoes and season to taste again.

SPICY POTATOES: INGREDIENTS FOR 2 SERVINGS:

Crystal salt
550 g small potatoes
1 teaspoon marjoram
2 tbsp coconut oil
1 pinch of chilli flakes
300 ml vegetable broth
1 teaspoon paprika, noble sweet

PREPARATION:

Wash, peel and dice the potatoes. Heat the oil in a pan. Fry the potatoes
in it for 3–5 minutes. Season to taste with the spices. Then deglaze the
potatoes with the vegetable stock. Let everything cook for about 15
minutes and stir occasionally.

FRUITY KOHLRABI SALAD: INGREDIENTS FOR 2 SERVINGS:

1 handful of chopped parsley
1 large kohlrabi
1-2 tbsp lemon juice
1 apple
2 tbsp olive oil
2 parsnips
6 tbsp oat cream
1 small piece of ginger

PREPARATION:

Peel and roughly grate the kohlrabi and parsnips. Roughly grate the apple
and drizzle with the lemon juice. Finely grate the ginger. Mix all
ingredients together. Let the salad stand for 15 minutes. Then season again
to taste and serve.

SPRING-LIKE, COLORFUL SALAD: INGREDIENTS FOR 4 SERVINGS:

2 carrots
1 bunch of dandelions
1/2 stick of leek
1 bunch of rocket
1/2 bunch of wild garlic
1 bunch of radishes with leaves
1/2 bunch Postelein

PREPARATION:

Wash and drain the radish leaves, dandelions, wild garlic, rocket and Postelein. Cut everything into small pieces. Wash the radishes and cut into thin slices. Wash the leek and cut into rings. Peel the carrots and cut into chips. Mix everything together.

CAULIFLOWER PAN: INGREDIENTS FOR 2 SERVINGS:

1/2 teaspoon cumin
1 small cauliflower
1/2 teaspoon ginger powder
150 g mustard sprouts
1/2 teaspoon turmeric
2 cloves of garlic
100 ml coconut milk
1 onion
2 tbsp coconut oil
1 bunch of parsley
125 ml vegetable broth without yeast

PREPARATION:

Separate the florets from the cauliflower. Chop the onion and garlic. Heat the coconut oil in a pan and sauté the onion and garlic. Then add the cauliflower. Deglaze everything with the vegetable stock and bring to the boil. Close the pan with a lid and simmer the cauliflower for 5 minutes over medium heat. Then add the sprouts, turmeric, ginger, salt, cumin, pepper and coconut milk. Let everything thicken while stirring constantly. Chop the parsley and pour over the cauliflower.

DESSERTS: APPLE DESSERT

Ingredients for 4 persons:
cinnamon

2 ripe quinces
ground vanilla
250 ml of water
200 g whippable soy cream
80 g stevia
1 teaspoon honey
2 tbsp lemon juice
2 apples

PREPARATION:

First the quinces are rubbed vigorously with a cloth. Then they are peeled, quartered and cut into cubes. The water is boiled with the stevia and lemon juice. Reduce the stevia-lemon water a little and then add the quince cubes. These should cook in the water. The apples are roughly grated and mixed with the honey and lemon juice. Then the apples are seasoned with vanilla and cinnamon. The soy cream is whipped until stiff and half of the cream is folded into the apple mixture. Now the apple cream is divided between 4 glass plates. The quince cubes are drained and added to the apple cream. The rest of the cream is poured over it to decorate.

FRUITY DREAM: INGREDIENTS FOR 2 PEOPLE:

250 g of grapes
2 teaspoons of cornstarch
1 ripe banana
100 ml red fruit juice
2 tsp stevia
150 g fresh or frozen raspberries

PREPARATION:

The cornstarch is stirred with 2 tablespoons of red fruit juice until smooth. The remaining fruit juice is put in a saucepan with the raspberries and brought to the boil. Then the whole thing is simmered for 4–5 minutes on low heat. The mixed cornstarch is now added to the berries and boiled while stirring. Now the stevia is stirred in. Let the berries simmer for about 1 minute and then pour them through a sieve. Strain the berries through the sieve. The bananas are peeled and cut into small cubes. These are mixed into the berry sauce. Finally, the grapes are washed and plucked from the stems and set aside to drain. Then the banana and berry sauce is spread over two dessert plates. The grapes are served on the dessert.

CINNAMON CREAM WITH APPLES: INGREDIENTS FOR 10 PEOPLE:

some lemon balm leaves
1 kg of apples
Juice of one lemon
100 g raisins
250 g whippable soy cream
100 ml apple juice
1/2 teaspoon ground cinnamon
80 g stevia
250 g natural yogurt

PREPARATION:

First the apples are peeled and cored. Then they are quartered and cut into thin slices. The apple slices are placed in a saucepan. Together with the raisins, apple juice, lemon juice and stevia, the apple slices are cooked in the pan for about 5 minutes. The apples should be firm to the bite. Then take the pot off the stove and let it cool down. In the meantime, stir the yogurt with the cinnamon. The cream is whipped until stiff and folded into the yoghurt cream. The cooled apple pieces are distributed on dessert bowls. The cinnamon cream is given over it. For serving, the dessert can be garnished with lemon balm.

BLUEBERRY MUFFINS: INGREDIENTS FOR 12 PIECES:

12 paper muffin cases

200 g whole wheat flour
2 tbsp water
60 g of oatmeal
300 g of oat cream
2 teaspoons of baking soda
180 g stevia
1/2 teaspoon baking soda
2 eggs
250 g blueberries

PREPARATION:

The oven is preheated to 160 ° C. The muffin tin is laid out with the baking molds. Now the flour is mixed with the oat flakes, baking soda and baking powder. The blueberries are cleaned and washed. Then the eggs are whisked and mixed with the stevia, water and oat cream. Now the flour mixture is folded in. Finally, add the blueberries. Pour the finished dough into the muffin molds and bake in the preheated oven for 20-25 minutes. As soon as the baking time is up, take the muffins out of the oven and let them rest for 5 minutes.
Tip: The muffins can also be frozen.

STUFFED COCONUT FIGS: INGREDIENTS FOR 10 PIECES:

10 whole pecans
10 dried figs
10 teaspoons of raw almond butter
1/4 cup fresh desiccated coconut
Preparation:
First the figs are cut lengthways and filled with the almond butter. The filled figs are rolled out in the desiccated coconut and decorated with a pecan nut.

MACADAMIA AND ALMOND CREAM: INGREDIENTS:

1 kg of fresh cherries

300 g macadamia nuts
1/2 teaspoon stevia (more or less depending on your taste)
60 g almonds
1 tbsp vanilla powder
2 cups of fresh almond milk

PREPARATION:

The macadamia nuts and almonds are soaked in water for at least 12 hours. The soaked nuts are now put in a blender. Stevia, almond milk and vanilla powder are added and mixed together until a creamy consistency is obtained. If the consistency is too firm, some almond milk can be added. Now the cream has to rest in the refrigerator for at least 3 hours. The finished cream is served with the cherries.

ESPRESSO COCOA DELICACY: INGREDIENTS FOR 2 SERVINGS:

1 banana
200 ml of sweet whey
50 ml espresso
1 pinch of cocoa
2 teaspoons of cocoa
1 pk. vanilla sugar

PREPARATION:: PREPARE ESPRESSO AND LET IT COOL DOWN.

Then bananas, whey, vanilla sugar and cocoa are combined and mashed. Stir in the espresso and serve with a drinking straw.

COCONUT COOKIES: INGREDIENTS FOR 10 COOKIES:

150 g coconut flakes
2 ripe bananas
Preparation:
Mash the bananas, add the coconut flakes and stir together. Preheat the

oven to 150 ° C. Shape the mixture into cookies and spread them on a baking sheet lined with baking paper. Bake the cookies for 15–20 minutes.

COCONUT CHEESECAKE: INGREDIENTS FOR AN 18 CM SPRINGFORM PAN:

For the ground:
cinnamon
1 banana
6 tbsp ground tiger nuts
For the crowd:
2 bananas
200 g Creamed Coconut

PREPARATION:

First preheat the oven to 170 ° C. Mash the banana for the bottom. Mix in the tiger nuts and some cinnamon. Line the springform pan with baking paper. Spread the banana mixture on the bottom of the springform pan. Bake the finished base for 20-25 minutes. Then let the base cool down. Now set the oven to 100 ° C. Let the creamed coconut soften in a container in the oven. Puree the mixture with the bananas in a blender. Spread the mixture on the cake base and let it harden in the refrigerator.

CARROT CAKE: INGREDIENTS FOR A CAKE: (BAKING PAN 20 X 20 CM)

For the cake:
2 tbsp coconut oil
3 carrots
1/2 teaspoon cinnamon
2 bananas
170 g desiccated coconut
140 g ground almonds
For the topping:
1/2 tbsp coconut oil
150 g white almond butter

25 ml of water
25 ml lime juice

PREPARATION:

Puree the bananas and carrots. Heat the coconut oil in a saucepan. Mix the banana mixture with the almonds, desiccated coconut, cinnamon and coconut oil. Put everything in the baking pan. Mix the almond butter with the water, the lime juice and the liquid coconut oil. Spread the whole thing on the cake. Let the finished cake set in the refrigerator for at least 1 hour.

FRUIT ICE CREAM: INGREDIENTS FOR 4 SERVINGS:

1 tbsp almond butter
1 avocado
100 ml orange juice
1 mango
1 banana

Preparation:

Core the avocado. Remove the pulp and cut into small pieces. Peel the mango and the banana and cut them into small pieces. Freeze everything for a few hours. Let the frozen fruits thaw and mix together with the orange juice and almond butter until creamy.

CUP APPLE PIE: INGREDIENTS FOR 1 CAKE:

1/2 cup raisins
1 cup of ground walnuts
1/2 cup desiccated coconut
1 cup of dates
1/2 cup of fresh apple juice
1/2 cup of raw sunflower seeds
2 1/2 teaspoons of cinnamon
4 cups of grated apples

PREPARATION:

Soak the dates and sunflower seeds in alkaline water, the dates for 15 minutes and the sunflower seeds for 20 minutes. Mix 2/3 of the coconut flakes with the drained dates, sunflower seeds and walnuts. Put the mixture in a cake tin. Mix the grated apples with the cinnamon, apple juice and raisins. Put the apple mixture on the cake base and sprinkle the remaining desiccated coconut on top.

HEARTY GRANOLA BARS: INGREDIENTS FOR 10 BARS:

1/4 teaspoon chili powder
500 g sunflower seeds
1/2 tsp organic coriander powder
1 red pepper
1 teaspoon sea salt
2 celery stalks
2 heaped teaspoons of organic paprika powder
1/2 onion
1 bunch of parsley
1 handful of young spinach leaves
1 teaspoon of minced garlic

PREPARATION:

Soak the sunflower seeds in 120 ml of water overnight. Wash, core and cut the bell peppers. Chop the celery, onion, spinach and parsley as well. Chop the vegetables in a blender. Then add the sunflower seeds and mix again. Shape the mixture into bars and bake in the oven on low heat.

DATE PRALINES: INGREDIENTS FOR 24 PRALINES:

100 g unsweetened desiccated coconut
2 cups of fresh dates
80 ml of water

Preparation:

Bring the dates to the boil with the water and stir occasionally until a paste is formed. Let the mixture cool down and shape into balls. Roll these in the coconut flakes and let them cool in the refrigerator.

DATE SMOOTHIE: INGREDIENTS:

fresh cinnamon
2 fresh dates
1 cup of fresh, chilled coconut milk
Preparation:
Puree the coconut milk with the dates and cinnamon in a blender.

ALMOND AND COCONUT WEDGES: INGREDIENTS:

Juice of half a lemon
200 ml of liquid coconut oil
200 g fresh coconut flakes
220 g of chopped almonds

PREPARATION:

Soak the almonds in water overnight. Then mix all ingredients except for 50 g desiccated coconut. Put the mixture in a baking dish. Sprinkle the remaining desiccated coconut on top. Let everything cool in the refrigerator for about 1 hour. Then cut small pieces out of the mass.

STRAWBERRY PUDDING: INGREDIENTS FOR 2 SERVINGS:

some chopped pistachios
2 tbsp chia seeds
180 g strawberries
100 ml of plant milk
2 tsp stevia
1 teaspoon lemon juice

PREPARATION:

Mix the milk with the chia seeds, lemon juice and 1 teaspoon stevia. Let it soak for at least 2 hours. Stir several times. Put 4–5 strawberries aside. Puree the remaining strawberries with 1 teaspoon stevia. Halve the remaining strawberries and chop the pistachios. Stir the swollen chia seeds once more and layer them in glasses with the strawberry puree. Place the halved strawberries on top.

APPLE-CREAM: INGREDIENTS FOR 2 SERVINGS:

250 g lupine yogurt
360 g apple pulp
1 tbsp lemon juice
4 heaped teaspoons of ground brown millet
1 teaspoon cinnamon
2 heaped tbsp tiger nuts flakes

PREPARATION:: MIX ALL INGREDIENTS AND STIR WELL.

Avocado Mousse
Ingredients for 4 persons:
1 1/2 teaspoons of sea salt
2 avocados
5 dates
200 ml coconut water
2 tbsp raw cocoa
1 tbsp vanilla

PREPARATION:

Stone the avocados and remove the pulp. Mix the pulp with the remaining ingredients. Let the mass solidify in the refrigerator for 4 hours.

STRAWBERRY AND AVOCADO CREAM: INGREDIENTS FOR 2 SERVINGS:

2 ripe avocados
250 g ripe strawberries
1 tbsp agave syrup
2 tbsp coconut oil
For the decoration:
Strawberries
Coconut flakes
Mint leaves

PREPARATION:

Stone the avocados and remove the pulp. Cut the pulp into slices. Wash the strawberries and mix together with the avocado, coconut oil and agave syrup. Pour the cream into bowls and garnish with some strawberries, the mint leaves and the coconut flakes.

Chapter Two

WHAT IS RHEUMATISM?

*E*veryone has probably felt the symptoms at some point: the joints hurt, functionality is limited, the symptoms come and go. Sometimes they only appear occasionally, but for many affected, every movement becomes increasingly torture. The suspicion quickly arises that one might suffer from rheumatism. The correct medical name is rheumatoid arthritis, but what does it mean? Which factors favor the occurrence of the symptoms and how can you, as the person affected, help to alleviate the symptoms? Once rheumatism is diagnosed, you will of course receive excellent care from your doctor. But you can also make a big contribution to improvement through an adequate diet. So what do you need to know about rheumatism and proper nutrition, and what is an anti-inflammatory diet? Rheumatism is a disease of the joints. They are caused by inflammation and, over time, cause pain and decrease in joint function. This simultaneously reduces mobility, which ultimately leads to a deterioration in quality of life. If the disease is not treated, the joints can even be destroyed in the long term. That is why an early diagnosis with the right medication is so important.

Doctors assume that around one percent of the population suffers from rheumatism, with women more often affected than men. Between the ages of 55 and 64, the disease is diagnosed particularly often in women; in men, it is more likely to be diagnosed from the age of 65. It is characteristic of the joints to function quickly and quickly as soon as the disease has reached a stage in which it can be identified. Rheumatism is basically an autoimmune disease. This means that the immune system turns against your own body and thereby damages it. The actual cause of the disease has not yet been researched, but scientists assume that a genetic defect could have a major impact. If there is already a genetic predisposition, the disease can easily be triggered by environmental factors. The activity of the immune system in rheumatism is primarily directed against a wide variety of joints. The cells of the immune system attack the synovium and the articular cartilage, causing inflammation in the joint itself. The synovium thickens more and more and is replaced by a type of connective tissue. This greatly affects the normal function of the joint. Over time, the joint becomes stiff and loses its functionality. Typical symptoms of rheumatism are swelling with pain in the joints. Usually the smaller joints on the hand, fingers and toes are affected first. A certain morning stiffness is also noticeable, it occurs after getting up and lasts for several hours. During this time, the joints feel heavier so that you can only move slowly. In addition to the joints, the bursa or tendons are also affected by the inflammation.

Inflammatory diseases of a chronic nature are becoming more and more important in our modern world. Already in ancient times it was recognized that diseases and ailments of various kinds influence each other through a suitable diet. As such chronic diseases are becoming more and more important today, it is good to know how you can help yourself through an adapted lifestyle. Doctors and inflammation researchers assume that our genetic makeup has not changed significantly over the centuries. So there must be other factors that are the cause of inflammatory diseases in the body and that did not previously exist in this form. Inflammation researchers in particular assume that nutrition is of enormous importance. It is said to be responsible for many ailments, because many doctors, scientists and nutritionists believe that our modern eating habits are not healthy.

If you suffer from rheumatism, you should get used to a diet that reduces the inflammatory processes in the body. Basically, inflammation in the body is an important process because it enables the immune system to defend itself against bacteria, fungi or viruses. If these inflammations are chronic, however, they attack the body's own tissue. Inflammation of the joints is just one example of the following disease, but ultimately they play a role in very different complaints. But how can you influence your rheumatism with the right diet?

WHAT IS OSTEOARTHRITIS?

Osteoarthritis is a disease of the joints. Whenever we move, we use our joints. A transparent cartilage between the bones ensures that they do not rub against each other with every movement. Joint fluid from the joint capsules supplies the cartilage with sufficient nutrients. The less we move, the less synovial fluid is produced. As a result, there are signs of wear and tear on the joints, which in medicine are referred to as osteoarthritis. In most cases, the hip or knee joints are affected, but finger and ankle joints also run the risk of wearing out with increasing age.

Chapter Three

BASIC RULES OF NUTRITION

*P*ay attention to the season: Common sense should already be aware that strawberries in winter must be imported or stored. Likewise, papayas will not be grown by local farmers even in summer. Be aware that seasonal and regionally available fruit and vegetables contain the most micronutrients and pay attention to what ends up in your shopping cart when shopping.

Number of servings: While our ancestors still mainly fed on fruit, vegetables and herbs, in the age of abundance, foods rich in fat and sugar are increasingly replacing healthy plants and fruits. According to the German Nutrition Society, around five servings of fruit and vegetables should be consumed every day. This recommendation should be followed, especially in the case of osteoarthritis. To do this, simply have a handful of fruit or vegetables with each meal.

Provide variety: It may be that you get all your nutrients optimally covered by a perfectly planned menu, but if you have to eat the same food for weeks, you will quickly fall back into old behavior patterns. Therefore, try out new recipes and ingredients every now and then and add a little variety to your diet.

Look for alternatives: Especially at the beginning of the diet change, you will miss one or the other food on the menu. So make a list right at the beginning of how you can replace unsuitable foods with healthy ones. Instead of wheat rolls, for example, eat whole-grain rolls if you don't want to do without your rolls at all, or choose the low-fat variant for dairy products.

Don't skimp on spices: since fat is a flavor carrier, you have to come up with something so that your dishes don't taste bland. Experiment with a variety of spices until you come up with a mix that comforts you over the lack of fat. However, be careful not to consume too much salt. The average German already consumes significantly more than the recommended 6 g of salt per day.

Eat mindfully: Various studies show that slim people often take more time to eat. Those who eat consciously and do not distract themselves with television or smartphone at the same time perceive the different tastes much more intensely. Chips suddenly don't taste that good anymore if they are eaten slowly and with full attention. Only now do you notice how greasy and unappetizing the little fattening foods actually are.

BREAKFAST: BLUEBERRY QUINOA

Ingredients for 2 people:
1/2 teaspoon vanilla extract
50 g raisins
1 cup of quinoa
1 teaspoon cinnamon powder
1 small apple, cut into cubes
750 ml unsweetened almond milk
1 cup blueberries (alternatively raspberries or strawberries)
1 handful of sunflower seeds
Apple syrup
1 handful of walnuts

PREPARATION:

First, put the quinoa in a saucepan with the almond milk and cinnamon. After that, everything is brought to a boil. As soon as the contents boil, the pot is covered. Now the stove is put on a low flame so that the contents simmer gently. Stir everything well from time to time so that nothing burns. After everything has simmered again for 5 minutes, the apple cubes and the raisins are added. Then everything has to simmer again for 5 minutes. After the 5 minutes have elapsed, the pot is removed from the stove so that the contents can be drawn with the lid closed. Now everything is seasoned with the apple syrup and the berries and nuts are stirred in. Then the blueberry quinoa can be served.

MUESLI WITH CRUNCH: INGREDIENTS FOR 2 PEOPLE:

2 dates
2 ripe bananas
Juice of half a lemon
2 apples
1 tbsp agave syrup
4 teaspoons of tiger nuts
6 walnut halves

PREPARATION:

First the bananas and apples are peeled. The bananas are then cut into slices and the apples into small pieces. The cut fruit is put aside in a bowl. The dates are also cut into small pieces and the walnut halves roughly chopped. Now the roughly chopped walnut halves are placed in a coated pan with the agave syrup and briefly roasted. Then the walnut halves are mixed into the fruit together with the tiger nut flakes, lemon juice and dates.

THE FRUITY BOMB: INGREDIENTS FOR 2 PEOPLE:

1/2 pineapple
1 pear
2 kiwis
2 carrots

Preparation:

The pineapple is peeled and cut into pieces. The pieces should fit in a juicer later. The carrots are brushed with a vegetable brush under running water and also cut into pieces for the juicer. Likewise, the kiwi is peeled and cut into pieces if necessary. The pear is washed and pitted thoroughly. Then it is cut into coarse cutlets. Now the fruit juice is pressed with the juicer. Fill this into a glass and enjoy the fruity bomb.

PORRIDGE WITH TIGER NUTS: INGREDIENTS FOR 1 PERSON:

1 teaspoon of crushed flaxseed
4 tbsp organic tiger nut flakes
2 dried, unsulphurized figs
100 ml hot spring water (alternatively hot almond milk)
1/2 apple
1 banana

PREPARATION:

The tiger nut flakes are poured over with hot water, stirred and set aside to swell. In the meantime, the banana can be peeled and mashed with a fork. The apple is washed and finely grated. The figs are also cut into small pieces. Finally, the mashed bananas, the grated apple and the figs are added to the tiger nut flake porridge together with the flaxseed. For serving, the porridge is arranged in a bowl.

PORRIDGE WITH APPLE: INGREDIENTS FOR 1 SERVING:

cardamom
3 tbsp buckwheat
1 apple
2 tbsp oatmeal
cinnamon
2 tbsp almonds
unsweetened grain drink (oats, almonds or spelled)

PREPARATION:

The almonds are roughly chopped and soaked in a little water with the buckwheat overnight and then rinsed through a sieve the next day. The almonds and buckwheat are now put in a saucepan with the grain drink and oat flakes. Everything is heated on a low flame with the pot closed. In the meantime, the apple is grated and can be added to the porridge. Finally, season everything with cardamom and cinnamon and serve warm.

PORRIDGE WITH COCONUT AND RASPBERRIES: INGREDIENTS FOR 2 PEOPLE:

salt
150 g raspberries
6 tbsp oatmeal
150 g red currants
350 ml coconut milk
50 g desiccated coconut
1 tbsp rice syrup

PREPARATION:

First the good raspberries and currants are sorted out. After that, they are washed, carefully patted dry and placed in a bowl. Now the raspberries and currants are mixed together and set aside. The coconut milk is put in a saucepan with the oat flakes, desiccated coconut and a pinch of salt. Bring everything to the boil while stirring. Then the porridge is taken off the stove to cool down. For serving, the porridge is layered alternately with the berry mixture in a glass. If you want, you can garnish everything with mint leaves.

GINGER AND CUCUMBER SMOOTHIE: INGREDIENTS FOR 1 SERVING:

1 tbsp linseed oil
1/2 cucumber
2 handfuls of lamb's lettuce
Water ad libitum
2–3 tart apples
1 piece of ginger, finger length
1 handful of romaine lettuce

PREPARATION:

First the fruit, the cucumber and the lettuce leaves are washed. The apples are then quartered and pitted. The ginger is roughly chopped. All ingredients are then placed in a tall vessel and pureed with a hand blender or stand mixer.

OMELETTE WITH TOMATO: INGREDIENTS FOR 2 PEOPLE:

2 tbsp rapeseed oil
1 shallot
salt and pepper
100 g feta
2 tbsp mineral water
2 dried tomatoes
3 eggs
2 fresh tomatoes

PREPARATION:

The shallot is peeled and diced. The feta is crumbled and the dried tomatoes are cut into fine slices. The fresh tomatoes are washed, halved and pitted. Then they are cut into fine cubes. Now the eggs are whisked with salt, pepper and the mineral water. The oil is heated in a pan and the shallots are fried until golden. Then add the egg mixture and sprinkle with the crumbled feta and tomatoes. The egg must now set on a mild heat. Then the finished omelette can be halved and served on two plates.

NETTLE SEED LOW-FAT CURD: INGREDIENTS FOR 1 SERVING:

1 tbsp nettle seeds
1 tbsp wheat germ oil
75 g blueberries (fresh or frozen)
1 teaspoon rose hip powder
200 g low-fat quark

1 pinch of turmeric
1 tbsp flaxseed
1 tbsp linseed oil

PREPARATION:

The blueberries are rinsed and patted dry. Frozen blueberries must be thawed beforehand. The low-fat quark is stirred with the oil until smooth. The mixture can be made creamier with a little water if the oil is not enough as a liquid. The turmeric, rose hip powder and nettle seeds are now mixed into the low-fat quark. The blueberries are poured over it for serving.

OMELETTE WITH SMOKED SALMON: INGREDIENTS FOR 2 PEOPLE:

2 tbsp rapeseed oil
300 g cucumber
2 tbsp chives rolls
salt and pepper
2 tbsp dill, freshly chopped
1 box of garden cress
2 tbsp kefir
50 g smoked salmon
2 tbsp mineral water
3 eggs

PREPARATION:

The cucumbers are washed or peeled and cut diagonally into thin slices. Then the cucumber slices are laid out flat on a plate and sprinkled with salt. The salmon is cut into cubes and set aside. The cress is cut from the bed, washed and patted dry. The eggs are now whisked with salt, pepper, mineral water and the kefir. The dill and chives are lifted under the egg mixture. The oil is heated in a pan and the egg mixture is added. On low heat, the egg mixture must now set to an omelette. The diced salmon and cress are sprinkled over the omelette in the pan. This is now folded up, halved and served on the prepared cucumber slices on the plate. The finished omelette can be served immediately.

BANANA AND NUT MASH: INGREDIENTS FOR 1 SERVING:

1 tbsp linseed oil
30 g tiger nut flakes
30 ml coconut milk
1 banana
80 ml cashew milk

Preparation:

First mash the banana. Then mix in the tiger nuts flakes. Mix the whole thing with the coconut milk and cashew milk. Finally stir in the linseed oil.

APPLE AND NUT MUESLI: INGREDIENTS FOR 1 SERVING:

1 cup of lupine yogurt
1 apple
1 tbsp pumpkin seeds
2 tbsp tiger nut flakes
4 almonds
2 walnuts

Preparation:

Wash and dice the apple. Chop the walnuts and almonds. Mix both with the apple. Roast the pumpkin seeds in a pan without fat and add them to the apple. Then mix in the tiger nuts flakes. Finally, stir the whole thing with the lupine yoghurt.

FRUIT BOWL: INGREDIENTS FOR 1 SERVING:

2 tbsp hemp flour
1 avocado
1 banana
1 green apple

Preparation:

Halve the avocado and remove the stone. Puree the pulp of the avocado together with the banana. Then add the hemp flour and stir. Dice the apple and add it. Mix everything again.

APRICOT QUINOA PORRIDGE: INGREDIENTS FOR 3 SERVINGS:

1 tbsp pumpkin seeds
100 g quinoa
300 ml of oat milk
6 apricots
Preparation:
First wash and drain the quinoa. Bring the oat milk to the boil and cook the quinoa in it for about 10 minutes. In the meantime cut the apricots in half and remove the stones. Puree the pulp of the apricots. Put the finished quinoa in a bowl and mix with the pureed apricots. Finally, chop the pumpkin seeds and roast them in a pan without fat. Sprinkle these over the apricot quinoa porridge.

TIGERNUT PORRIDGE: INGREDIENTS FOR 1 SERVING:

1 pinch of cinnamon
60 g tiger nut flakes
1 teaspoon raw cocoa
100 ml rice milk
Preparation:
Bring the rice milk to the boil and stir in the tiger nuts flakes. Let the whole thing swell for about 10 minutes. Finally, season with the cocoa and cinnamon.

QUINOA PORRIDGE WITH CHERRIES: INGREDIENTS FOR 2 SERVINGS:

1 tbsp agave syrup
100 g quinoa
300 ml lupine drink
50 g frozen cherries
Preparation:

Bring the lupine drink to the boil in a saucepan. Then add the quinoa and simmer over medium heat for about 10 minutes. Then take the saucepan off the stove and add the frozen cherries. Finally, season the whole thing with the agave syrup.

ALMOND PANCAKES: INGREDIENTS FOR 1 SERVING:

Coconut oil
50 g almond flour
2 teaspoons coconut blossom sugar
20 g coconut flour
2 tbsp almond butter
20 g raw cocoa
200 ml almond milk

PREPARATION:

Mix the cocoa with the two types of flour. Then add the coconut blossom sugar and the almond milk and stir well. Heat the coconut oil in a pan and fry the dough in portions to make pancakes. Brush the finished pancakes with the almond butter.

RASPBERRY AND ALMOND MASH: INGREDIENTS FOR 1 SERVING:

1 teaspoon coconut blossom sugar
75 g quinoa
1 tbsp almond slicer
20 g ground almonds
50 ml of oat cream
50 g frozen raspberries
200 ml rice drink

PREPARATION:

Heat the rice drink in a saucepan. Let the quinoa simmer in it for about 10 minutes. Then stir in the ground almonds, oat cream and coconut blossom sugar. Let the whole thing swell briefly. Finally fold in the frozen raspberries and garnish with the almond slices.

NUT AND FRUIT MUESLI: INGREDIENTS FOR 1 SERVING:

1 cup of lupine yogurt
10 g of popped amaranth
10 g unsweetened banana chips
10g popped quinoa
10 g dried apples
10 g chopped almonds
10 g chopped walnuts

PREPARATION:

Mix all ingredients together except for the yoghurt. Finally add the yoghurt and stir everything together.

VEGETABLE AND FRUIT SMOOTHIE: INGREDIENTS FOR 1 SERVING:

1 teaspoon coconut blossom sugar
1 pear
100 ml almond milk
1 carrot

Preparation:

Peel and halve the pear. Then remove the core housing. Dice the carrot. Put the pear and carrot in a blender and puree. Then add the almond milk and mix everything again. Season the smoothie with the coconut blossom sugar.

FRUIT YOGURT DRINK: INGREDIENTS:

1 tbsp coconut butter
1 banana

100 g lupine yogurt
50 g sour cherries
100 ml rice drink

Preparation:

Peel and cut the banana. Core the cherries and remove the stems. Put both in a blender and puree. Then add the rice drink and coconut butter and mix again. Finally add the yoghurt.

ORANGE SMOOTHIE: INGREDIENTS:

250 ml almond milk
1 peach
4 apricots

Preparation:

Wash the fruit and cut in half. Remove the stones and seeds. Then puree the fruit and add the almond milk. Mix the whole thing well together again.

ALMOND AND FRUIT SMOOTHIE: INGREDIENTS:

1 teaspoon almond butter
1 apple
100 ml almond milk
100 g sweet cherries

Preparation:

Wash the fruit and remove the stones and stems. Cut the apple into small pieces and puree with the cherries. Then add the almond milk and almond butter and mix everything together again.

YEAST-FREE SPELLED BREAD: INGREDIENTS FOR 1 BREAD:

olive oil
500 g spelled flour (type 630)
100 g pumpkin seeds
1/2 teaspoon salt
100 g of flaxseed

500 ml of lukewarm water
1 pk. Tartar baking powder
1 teaspoon bread spice mix

PREPARATION:

Mix the baking powder with the flour. Then mix in the bread spices, flax seeds and pumpkin seeds. Then add the water and knead everything together. Brush a loaf pan with the olive oil and pour in the batter. Then brush the surface of the dough again with a little water. Bake the bread for 60 minutes at 200 ° C top / bottom heat.

FRUIT PULP WITH POMEGRANATE SEEDS: INGREDIENTS FOR 2 SERVINGS:

1 pomegranate
100 g buckwheat
100 ml almond milk
2 pears
2 teaspoons of lemon juice
1 banana
2 tsp almond butter
1 apple
2 teaspoons of sweet lupine flour as required
1 handful of raisins

PREPARATION:

Soak the buckwheat in water for 1 hour. Then pour through a sieve and rinse. So that the buckwheat can germinate, place the sieve over a bowl and rinse under water in the morning and evening. As soon as the buckwheat sprouts, place 3–4 tablespoons on a baking sheet and leave to dry in the oven at 50 ° C for approx. 3–4 hours. Put the remaining buckwheat with the flour, lemon juice, raisins and almond butter and almond milk in a blender. Remove the core from the apple and pears. Cut all the fruit into small pieces and add to the buckwheat mixture. Mix everything well. If the porridge is too firm, it can be diluted with a little almond milk. Remove the seeds from the pomegranate. Put the finished porridge in a bowl and spread the pomegranate seeds and the cooled buckwheat kernels on top.

FRUIT CEREAL: INGREDIENTS FOR 1 SERVING:

2–3 tbsp oat flakes (alternatively granola)
1 small banana
some blueberries
1 tart apple
1 juice orange

PREPARATION:

First squeeze the orange. Cut the banana into slices and mix carefully with the orange juice. Wash the apple and cut into small cubes. Mix the apple with the blueberries into the banana. Finally fold in the oatmeal.

FRUIT PORRIDGE: INGREDIENTS FOR 1 SERVING:

1 handful of fresh fruit (alternatively dried fruit)
3–4 tablespoons of glued oat flakes
1 teaspoon chopped almonds
100 ml coconut milk
1 teaspoon sesame seeds
1 pinch of salt

PREPARATION:

Heat the coconut milk and stir in the oatmeal. Then simmer the porridge for about 3–5 minutes over low heat. Remove the pan from the heat and season the porridge with the salt. Cut the fruit into small pieces and fold into the pulp.

BANANA MASH: INGREDIENTS FOR 1 SERVING:

Vanilla or cinnamon
300 ml almond milk
1 banana
4 tbsp ground tiger nuts
2 tbsp lupine protein vanilla

PREPARATION:

In a saucepan, bring the almond milk with the lupine protein and the tiger nuts to the boil. Let it simmer for 5–7 minutes. During this time, mash the banana. Fold the mashed banana into the pulp. Finally, season the whole thing with vanilla or cinnamon.

APRICOT AND CINNAMON PORRIDGE: INGREDIENTS FOR 2 SERVINGS:

1 pinch of salt
120 g millet
1/3 teaspoon cinnamon
150 ml coconut milk
2 tbsp ground flaxseed
200 ml of water
1 tbsp sesame seeds
1 apple
2 tbsp coconut flakes
4 dried, unsulphurized apricots

PREPARATION:

First wash and rinse the millet. Bring the coconut milk, water, sesame, linseed, millet and salt to the boil. In the meantime, wash the apple and remove the core. Cut the pulp into pieces and add to the coconut milk. Chop the apricots and stir in. Let it simmer over a low heat for 5–6 minutes. Then put everything aside for about 10 minutes to swell. Toast the coconut flakes in a pan without oil. Finally fold in the coconut flakes and cinnamon.

GREEN VEGETABLE SMOOTHIE: INGREDIENTS FOR 1 SERVING:

6–8 ice cubes
1 avocado
1 pk. Stevia
1/2 English cucumber
1 teaspoon of super green powder
1 small tomato
2 teaspoons of bean sprouts powder
1 lime
2 cups of fresh spinach

PREPARATION:: FIRST PEEL THE LIME. HALVE THE AVOCADO AND REMOVE THE STONE. PUT EVERYTHING IN A BLENDER AND MIX.

Spicy smoothie
Ingredients:
Ice cubes
1 small cucumber
1 pinch of salt and pepper
1 stick of celery
1/2 chilli pepper
4 Roma tomatoes
1 lemon (alternatively 2 limes)

PREPARATION:

Cut the vegetables into small pieces and puree them in a blender. Squeeze the juice from the lemon and add to the vegetables. Chop the chilli pepper and add it along with salt and pepper. Mix everything again. Fill ice cubes in glasses and distribute the smoothie in them.

VEGETABLE JUICE: INGREDIENTS:

3 carrots
1 medium-sized cucumber
1 medium beetroot
1 green pepper
2 tomatoes

Preparation:

Cut the vegetables into small pieces and squeeze out the juice with a
juicer. The vegetable juice can be diluted with water.

VEGETABLE AND MINT SMOOTHIE: INGREDIENTS FOR 1 SERVING:

2-3 mint leaves
2 carrots
3 ice cubes
1 grapefruit
100 ml of pure water

Preparation:

Peel the carrots and grapefruit. Put both in a blender and puree. Dilute
the smoothie with the water and add the mint leaves.

TOFU SMOOTHIE WITH VEGETABLES: INGREDIENTS:

3-4 ice cubes
1 avocado
unsweetened soy milk
1 lime
1 handful of fresh spinach leaves
1 small cucumber

PREPARATION:

Halve the avocado and remove the stone. Then peel the avocado and lime. Cut the pulp of both into pieces. Cut the cucumber and tofu into cubes. Put everything in a blender and puree.

COCONUT FRUIT MUESLI: INGREDIENTS FOR 1 SERVING:

1 tbsp flaxseed
1 peach
1 tbsp quinoa sprouts
1 mandarin
30 g coconut flakes
Preparation:
Rinse the quinoa sprouts and flax seeds. Mix the coconut flakes with the almond milk. Wash and core the peach. Peel the tangerine. Cut this and the peach into small pieces. Finally mix everything together.

FRUIT MUESLI WITH CINNAMON: INGREDIENTS FOR 1 SERVING:

1 teaspoon carob powder
50 g fresh papaya
1 pinch of cinnamon
50 g fresh avocado
1 tbsp Chufas nuts
1 soaked fig
1-2 teaspoons acerola powder
1 soaked date
2-3 teaspoons of spirulina powder
1 small banana

PREPARATION:

Soak the dried fruits, then puree them with the soaking water, spirulina powder, carob powder, papaya and cinnamon. Put the Chufas nuts in a bowl and pour the dried fruit puree over it. Mix everything together well. Cut the banana into slices and sprinkle with the acerola powder. Finally mix everything again.

LEEKS: INGREDIENTS FOR 1 SERVING:

1 pinch of crystal salt
100 g tender leeks
1 pinch of miso
30 g buckwheat groats
5 g sunflower oil
8–10 tbsp vegetable broth without yeast (alternatively water)

PREPARATION:

Put the groats in boiling water while stirring and let swell over low heat. In the meantime, finely chop the leek and steam in a little water. Then mix the leek into the buckwheat groats and remove everything from the stove. Finally, season to taste with the oil, miso, vegetable stock and salt.

COLORFUL BREAKFAST PORRIDGE: INGREDIENTS FOR 1 SERVING:

some raisins or dried fruit
1 carrot
Walnuts as needed
1 apple
1 banana

Preparation:

Peel the carrot and apple. Remove the core from the apple. Cut the pulp of the apple, the carrot and the banana into large pieces. Puree all ingredients together.

PLUM SMOOTHIE WITH WALNUTS: INGREDIENTS FOR 2 SERVINGS:

250 ml of water
8 plums
40 ml of cherry juice
300 ml of water
4 teaspoons of flaxseed

1 banana

12 walnuts

PREPARATION:: SOAK THE PLUMS IN THE WATER. THEN PUREE ALL INGREDIENTS TOGETHER.

Main courses
Millet pancakes
Ingredients for 2–3 people:
Sea salt or organic salt

500 g millet

50 g sesame seeds

1 small carrot (alternatively 1/2 medium-sized carrot)

50 g sunflower seeds

1 1/2 onions

1 tbsp gluten-free soy flour

extra virgin, cold-pressed olive oil

PREPARATION:

Cut the onions and the carrot into small cubes. Put half a diced onion together with the carrot, millet and 1 teaspoon sea salt in 2 liters of water. Let everything simmer for about 40 minutes. Then put the cooked millet in a bowl and add the remaining onion that has already been diced. Also add the soy flour, sunflower seeds, sesame seeds and 1/2 teaspoon sea salt and mix everything together well. Now form a buffer from this. Heat some olive oil in a pan and gradually fry the buffers in it.

SAVOY CABBAGE POTATO PAN: INGREDIENTS FOR 4 PERSONS:

Vegetable broth

1 savoy cabbage

3 cloves of garlic

turmeric

1 red pepper

1 onion

1 large carrot

cumin
6 potatoes

PREPARATION:

The thick parts of the stalk are removed from the savoy cabbage leaves. The leaves are divided and then cut into strips. These are blanched in boiling salted water for 3 minutes. Dice the onion, potatoes, carrots and peppers and fry them in a pan with the flat-pounded garlic. Now deglaze the whole thing with 1/2 cup of water and steam with the lid closed for 5 minutes. After the 5 minutes have passed, add the savoy cabbage and season with vegetable stock, cumin and turmeric to taste. Mix everything together well and steam again for 5–10 minutes. It should be stirred again and again. If desired, sunflower seeds or pumpkin seeds can be added on top.

PASTA WITH ZUCCHINI AND EGGPLANT: INGREDIENTS FOR 2–3 PEOPLE:

Sea salt and freshly ground black pepper
300 g spelled pasta
2 tsp basil leaves, dried
1 large, diced aubergine (approx. 300 g)
1 teaspoon oregano
3 tbsp extra virgin olive oil
2/3 cup vegetable broth
1–2 finely diced, medium-sized onions
4 tbsp dried, diced tomatoes
3 medium, ripe, diced tomatoes
1 large, diced zucchini (approx. 400 g)

PREPARATION:

Heat the olive oil in a large pan. Fry the onions, garlic and aubergines for 8–10 minutes, stirring occasionally. Then the zucchini and all the tomatoes with the oregano are added and cooked again for 6–8 minutes. In between, the mass should be stirred so that nothing burns.

In the meantime, the spelled pasta is cooked al dente in water. Then the vegetable stock is added to the pan and everything is seasoned with salt, pepper and the dried basil. Let the pan simmer for a few minutes. To serve, the finished sauce is poured over the pasta.

VEGETABLE CURRY: INGREDIENTS FOR 2 SERVINGS:

Sea salt and fresh pepper
200 g carrots
1 tsp curry powder
250 g broccoli florets
100 ml of yeast-free vegetable stock
100 g peas
100 ml unsweetened coconut milk
1 tbsp oil
1 clove of garlic
1 medium onion

PREPARATION:

Chop the onion and garlic and set aside. The carrots are cut into slices and also set aside. In a pan or wok, heat the oil over a medium flame and sauté the onions, garlic and curry powder until translucent. Then add the carrot slices and broccoli florets and stir briefly. Then coconut milk and vegetable broth are added and everything is simmered on a low flame for 8-10 minutes with the lid closed. Every now and then everything should be stirred. Finally, season the whole thing with pepper, sea salt and a little lemon juice (if necessary). Bring everything to the boil again briefly and then serve.

RATATOUILLE: INGREDIENTS FOR 4 SERVINGS:

1 cup of water
5 tomatoes
1 pinch of cayenne pepper
1 large zucchini

1 pinch of sea salt (or organic salt)
1 large eggplant
3 tablespoons of cold-pressed, extra virgin olive oil
1 green pepper
2 tsp herbs from Provence (basil, marjoram, lavender, thyme, oregano, rosemary, sage)
1 large onion
2 cloves of garlic

PREPARATION:

The skin is removed from the peppers and tomatoes and the pulp is cut into cubes. The eggplant, onion, zucchini and garlic are cut into thin slices.
Put some olive oil in a pan or wok and heat. Sauté the onions and garlic for a few minutes. Then the zucchini slices, the diced paprika and the aubergine slices are added and sautéed for another 10 minutes. Occasionally everything should be stirred. Then the tomatoes, herbs and water are added and everything is mixed together well. Let it simmer again for a few minutes. Finally, the whole thing is seasoned with salt and pepper.

GREEK LENTIL SOUP: INGREDIENTS FOR 4 SERVINGS:

1/2 teaspoon oregano
300 g small, Greek lentils
1 bay leaf
2 fresh tomatoes
Sea salt and fresh pepper
1 carrot
1 tbsp fresh lemon juice
1/2 stick of leek
2 tablespoons of cold-pressed, extra virgin olive oil
1 onion
3-4 cloves of garlic

PREPARATION:

The lentils are washed well and soaked in plenty of water overnight. Drain the lentils the next day and simmer in hot water for 5 minutes. Then the lenses are poured off and drained again. The onion and cloves of garlic are finely chopped. Pureed the tomatoes and cut the carrots and leek into fine slices. Now put the tomato puree, the carrot slices, the onions, the chopped garlic cloves and the leek slices together with the bay leaf in 1/2 liter of water and bring to the boil over high heat. Then add the lentils and simmer gently over low heat for at least 30 minutes. It may be necessary to add some water. Finally, the olive oil and lemon juice are added and everything is seasoned with oregano, sea salt and pepper.

CELERY BROCCOLI SOUP: INGREDIENTS 2 SERVINGS:

salt and pepper
1 onion
0.5–1 liters of almond milk
1 head of celery
1–2 liters of vegetable stock
1 broccoli
Spices of your choice to taste
1 teaspoon oil

PREPARATION:

Chop the onion and fry in a little oil in a large stock pot for about 5 minutes. Cut the celery into pieces and set aside some of the leaves for garnish. Also cut the broccoli into small pieces and put in a blender along with the celery. Mix both ingredients until the vegetables are finely chopped. Add the celery and broccoli mix to the onions and heat. Then add the vegetable stock and the almond milk and simmer for about 15-30 minutes. Then puree the entire contents of the pot until a fine, creamy consistency is achieved. At the end everything is seasoned with salt and spices of your choice. The soup can be served warm or cold.

CHICKPEA SALAD WITH AVOCADO: INGREDIENTS FOR 2 PEOPLE:

3 spring onions
1 can of chickpeas
1 red pepper
1 handful of fresh spinach leaves
100 g asparagus (fresh or from the jar)
1 romaine lettuce
1 stick of celery
3 tomatoes
For the dressing:
1 pinch of sea salt
1 avocado
extra virgin, cold-pressed olive oil
Juice of one lemon

PREPARATION:

Except for the avocado, all ingredients are cut into small pieces and placed in a salad bowl. Then everything is mixed together well. Cut the flesh of the avocado into small pieces and place in a blender with the lemon juice and a little olive oil. Mix everything briefly until you have a thick dressing. If the dressing becomes too thick, a little water can be added. Pour the finished avocado salad dressing over the salad with a pinch of salt and mix everything together well.

STUFFED PEPPERS: INGREDIENTS FOR 2 SERVINGS:

sea-salt
1 large bell pepper (red or yellow)
1 large, ripe avocado
7 medium, fresh carrots
fresh herbs to taste

PREPARATION:

First, the peppers are washed, cut in half and both halves thoroughly cleaned. Then they can be put aside. The carrots are pressed through a juicer and processed into juicy pulp. Then the avocado is peeled and the pulp is pressed into the carrot puree with a fork. The carrot and avocado puree can now be seasoned with sea salt and the fresh herbs. At the end it is filled into the pepper halves and can be served.

AVOCADO SOUP: INGREDIENTS FOR 1 SERVING:

some water
1 avocado
1 pinch of sea salt
1 stick of celery
1 pinch of pepper
1 splash of fresh lemon juice
1 handful of fresh spinach
1 tomato

PREPARATION:

First the tomato is cut into small cubes. Then all the other ingredients are put in a blender and mashed on high. The finished soup can now be put in a soup bowl. Add the diced tomatoes and serve.

POTATO SALAD: INGREDIENTS FOR 4 PERSONS:

Salt and white pepper
1 kg of potatoes
3 tbsp oil
1/8 liter stock (instant)
1 bunch of radishes
4 tbsp herb vinegar
1 small stick of leek

PREPARATION:

First the potatoes are washed and then cooked for 20 minutes. Then the water is poured off and the potatoes can be peeled and put aside to cool. Once the potatoes have cooled, they are quartered and cut into pieces. Now pour the hot broth over the potato pieces and let it steep for 10 minutes. In the meantime, mix the herb vinegar, salt and pepper into a marinade. The potatoes are now mixed with the marinade. The whole thing now has to go through well again. Meanwhile, the leek is cleaned, washed and cut into fine rings. The radishes are also cleaned, washed and cut into fine slices. Before the potato salad is served, the radishes and leek are mixed with the oil with the salad.

VEGETABLE PAN WITH GARLIC DIP: INGREDIENTS FOR 2 PEOPLE:

For the pan:
Iodized salt and pepper
4 spring onions
fresh or dried herbs (oregano, thyme, rosemary)
2 carrots
1 tbsp olive oil
1 small zucchini
1 red pepper
For the dip:
Iodized salt and pepper
1 cup of yogurt, 1.5% fat
1 clove of garlic
2 tbsp sour cream
1 tbsp olive oil

PREPARATION:

First the vegetables are cleaned, washed and cut into fine strips. The olive oil is heated in a coated pan and the vegetables are added. Now the vegetables are cooked firm to the bite for about 15 minutes over medium

heat and often turned. Finally, the vegetable pan is seasoned with iodized
salt, pepper and the herbs.

For the dip:

Mix the yoghurt with the sour cream and the olive oil. The garlic clove is
squeezed out and also added. Finally, season the dip with salt and pepper.

SWISS CHARD LASAGNA: INGREDIENTS FOR 10-12 PEOPLE:

500 g of grated cheese
2.5 kg of Swiss chard
2.5 liters of vegetable stock
625 g mushrooms
7 tbsp flour
500 g onions
7 tbsp butter
1000 g lasagne sheets
7 tbsp oil

PREPARATION:

First the chard is cleaned and the green leaves are removed from the
stems. The stems are cut into short strips and the leaves are roughly
chopped. Everything is blanched in a saucepan with boiling water and
then drained. The mushrooms are cleaned and sliced. The onions are
diced and sweated in oil. Now the mushrooms and the chard are
added. With the lid closed, everything is steamed for about 10
minutes. The butter is melted and the flour is stirred in. The whole thing
is extinguished with the vegetable stock and briefly boiled. Now the sauce
is seasoned. Finally, the vegetables, the sauce and the lasagne sheets are
layered alternately in a baking dish. First the sauce and the last layer must
also be sauce. Sprinkle the lasagne with the grated cheese and bake at 170 °
C for 40 minutes.

BEETROOT SOUP: INGREDIENTS FOR 4 PERSONS:

salt

500 g beetroot
100 ml cream
1 onion
grated peel of an orange
2 carrots
750 ml vegetable stock
100 g potatoes
about 1 cm of ginger

PREPARATION:

First the beetroot and the onion are peeled and then diced. The carrots
and potatoes are brushed and also cut into cubes. The ginger is peeled and
grated. Sweat the onion cubes in oil and add the beetroot, carrots and
potatoes. The ginger is then added and everything is topped up with the
vegetable stock. Now the whole thing has to simmer for about 15
minutes. After the 15 minutes have elapsed, the contents of the pan are
pureed. Now everything has to be seasoned with salt and the grated
orange peel. Finally, the cream is whipped and drawn into the soup before
serving. As an alternative: Instead of ginger and orange peel, you can also
use some apple juice.

LIGHT PEA SOUP: INGREDIENTS FOR 4 PERSONS:

Salt and white pepper
2 pk. frozen peas (300 g each)
1/2 cup of whipped cream (100 g)
1 1/4 liters of clear broth
3 bunch of chervil / 3 eggs

PREPARATION:

Bring the peas together with the broth to the boil in a saucepan and cook
for about 15 minutes. Then the peas are finely pureed with the cutting
stick of the hand mixer. The eggs are placed in boiling water and hard-
boiled for 10 minutes, after which they are peeled off, cut in half and the

egg whites finely chopped. The chervil are washed thoroughly under running water and carefully shaken dry. Then some stalks are set aside and the rest are finely chopped. The egg white and chervil are added to the soup. Then the soup is seasoned with salt and pepper. The cream is slept stiffly and half drawn under the soup. The rest of the cream is given as a dollop on top of the soup for garnish. The egg yolk is now pressed through a fine press, for example a garlic press, and sprinkled over the soup together with the chervil that was set aside. Then the finished soup can be served.

CARROT SALAD WITH PINEAPPLE: INGREDIENTS FOR 2 PEOPLE:

4 large leaves of lettuce / 500 g carrots
2 tbsp coconut flakes / 2 slices of pineapple
1 tbsp raisins
For the marinade: 1 pinch of cayenne pepper
3 tbsp lemon juice / 1 pinch of ground coriander
3 tbsp pineapple juice / 2 tbsp oil / 1 tbsp honey

PREPARATION:

First the carrots are finely grated. The pineapple is cut into small cubes and the raisins are washed. Everything is mixed together with the coconut flakes. For the marinade: Mix the lemon juice with the pineapple juice and honey. Then everything is seasoned with the cayenne pepper and the coriander and oil is added. The marinade is now mixed with the salad and placed in a cool place so that the salad can permeate well. Before serving, the salad should be seasoned again. For serving, the plates are covered with the lettuce leaves and the carrot salad is served on top.

BAKED CAULIFLOWER: INGREDIENTS FOR 4 PERSONS:

1 cup of crème fraîche, 1.5 fat (150 g)
2 small heads of cauliflower
2 egg yolks
salt

1/2 teaspoon ground nutmeg
Fat for the shape
1 pk. Peas (300 g)
1 tsp curry
30 g butter or margarine
1/2 liter of almond milk
30 grams of flour

PREPARATION:

The cauliflower is cleaned, washed and cut into small florets. Then the florets are blanched for 5 minutes in boiling salted water. 1/2 liter of the cauliflower water is poured off through a sieve and stored. Put the cauliflower florets and the peas in a greased baking dish. Fat is heated for the sauce. The flour is sweated in it and then extinguished with the almond milk and the cauliflower water. Now the whole thing has to boil again, the sauce is seasoned with salt, curry and nutmeg. The egg yolk is mixed with the crème fraîche and stirred into the sauce. This is now poured over the vegetables in the baking dish and baked for 35-40 minutes at 200 ° C (electric stove). On a gas stove, the casserole is baked on level 3. If you want, you can serve mashed potatoes with it.

ZUCCHINI STEW: INGREDIENTS FOR 3 PEOPLE:

pepper from the grinder
40 g margarine
1/8 liter of water
2 onions
1 pinch of saffron
300 g zucchini
1 teaspoon oregano
1 small savoy cabbage
2 teaspoons of herbal salt
1 leek
50 g grated Gouda cheese
250 g tomatoes

PREPARATION:

Peel the onions and cut into rings. Steam the onion rings in a pan with fat until translucent. Cut the zucchini into slices, the savoy cabbage into strips and the leek into rings. Then the vegetables are added to the onions and sautéed briefly. Now the water is added and everything is cooked for 20 minutes. In the meantime, peel the tomatoes, cut them in half and add them to the pan after 10 minutes. In addition, everything is seasoned with herbal salt, pepper, saffron and oregano. Just before the dish is served, sprinkle everything with cheese and parsley. Crispy farmer's bread can be served with it.

CELERY AND APPLE RAW VEGETABLES: INGREDIENTS FOR 4 PERSONS:

1 tbsp chopped hazelnuts
250 g celeriac
1 lettuce
250 g sour apples
4 teaspoons of lemon juice
1 cup of skimmed milk yogurt (175 g)

PREPARATION:

Wash and then peel the celery and apples. The apples are quartered and pitted. The celery is cut into pieces. Then both ingredients are grated and immediately drizzled with lemon juice. The skimmed milk yogurt is stirred until smooth. The lettuce is washed, drained and the leaves are distributed on four plates. Spread the raw vegetables on the lettuce leaves and put a blob of yogurt per serving on top. The hazelnut kernels are then sprinkled over the top.

PEA SOUP WITH DUMPLINGS: INGREDIENTS FOR 4 PERSONS:

1/2 teaspoon salt
2 kg of fresh green peas

grated nutmeg
2 onions
1 bunch of parsley
75 g margarine
2 eggs
4 tbsp chicken broth
125 g spelled flour
1/4 liter of milk

PREPARATION:

The peas are first peeled, rinsed and drained. Now the onions are peeled
and finely diced. Approx. Heat 50 g of the margarine and sauté the onions
until translucent. Now the peas are added and steamed for 3 minutes. Now
the chicken broth is sprinkled in and extinguished with 1.5 liters of boiling
water. Let the soup simmer for 15 minutes. Now the milk, the salt and the
rest of the margarine are brought to the boil in a saucepan. The flour is
poured in and everything is stirred until it loosens from the bottom of the
pot as a lump. Now the pot is removed from the stove and the eggs are
gradually stirred into the batter. Now everything is seasoned. Small
dumplings are cut from the dough and carefully added to the soup. These
have to steep in the soup for 10 minutes. After that, everything is
sprinkled with chopped parsley.

HERBSOUP: INGREDIENTS FOR 4 PERSONS:

a few drops of lemon juice
50 g margarine
nutmeg
2 tbsp spelled flour
1 liter of almond milk
1 bunch each of chives, parsley, dill
3 teaspoons of condensed milk

PREPARATION:

First the margarine is heated in a saucepan. Then stir in the flour and sweat it until it has a golden yellow color. The almond milk is now poured on while stirring. Everything is left to cook for a few minutes. The herbs are finely chopped in the meantime. One half of the chopped herbs is added to the milk mass. This is also seasoned with, nutmeg and salt. The herb soup is now boiled until it has a creamy consistency. Then it is seasoned again and the remaining herbs and condensed milk are stirred in. Finally, the finished soup is seasoned with lemon juice.

COLESLAW: INGREDIENTS FOR 1 BOWL:

1 pinch of cayenne pepper
1/2 cabbage
1 cup coconut milk (preferably fresh coconut meat mixed with the coconut juice)
2 medium-sized carrots
2 tbsp extra virgin olive oil
1 small, red onion
1/2 tbsp fresh lemon juice
1/2 cup parsley
1/2 teaspoon sea salt

PREPARATION:

The parsley is finely chopped. The cabbage, carrots and onion are cut into fine strips. All ingredients are put in a bowl and mixed well there. The coconut milk is now spread over the salad and also mixed well with the other ingredients. The finished salad must now pull through well.

KALE SALAD: INGREDIENTS FOR 2 SERVINGS:

a bit of salt
250 g kale

2 tbsp lemon juice
200 g edamame
4 tbsp virgin olive oil
75 g dried cranberries
100 g cherry tomatoes

PREPARATION:

First wash the kale, remove the stem and shake dry. Then pluck the kale into bite-sized pieces. Mix the olive oil with the lemon juice and the salt and mix the kale with it. Let the whole thing stand in the refrigerator for about 10 minutes. In the meantime, bring the salted water to the boil and simmer the edamame for 3–4 minutes until soft. Then drain and rinse with cold water. Wash the cherry tomatoes and cut in half. Mix the kale with the tomatoes, edamame and cranberries and season the salad with salt and pepper.

CURRY POTATO PAN: INGREDIENTS FOR 2 PEOPLE:

2 tbsp sesame seeds
400 g potatoes
salt and pepper
400 g pointed cabbage
1/2 can of coconut milk
1 bell pepper
1 tsp curry
2 carrots
2 teaspoons of turmeric
2 tablespoons oil
2 onions

PREPARATION:

First wash the pointed cabbage and remove the stalk. Then cut the cabbage into fine strips. Cut the onions into fine cubes. Peel, wash and dice the potatoes and carrots. Wash, core and cut the peppers into strips. Heat the oil in a pan and fry the onions, potatoes and carrots in it for about 10 minutes. Then add the cabbage and fry everything for about 3 minutes. Deglaze the whole thing with the coconut milk and season with the spices. Bring everything to the boil and arrange on plates. Sprinkle the potato pan with the sesame seeds.

DUMPLINGS: INGREDIENTS FOR 2 PEOPLE:

nutmeg
6 potatoes
White pepper
4 sprigs of parsley
Seasoned Salt
3 teaspoons of virgin olive oil

Preparation:

Wash, peel and cut the potatoes. Cook the potato pieces in a steamer for about 15–20 minutes. In the meantime, wash the parsley and gently shake dry. Then pluck the leaves from the parsley and chop finely. Mash the finished potatoes into a pulp and mix with the olive oil, salt, nutmeg, pepper and parsley. Form dumplings from the mixture with two tablespoons and arrange them on plates.

POTATO AND KOHLRABI SOUP: INGREDIENTS FOR 2 PEOPLE:

parsley
5 kohlrabi
pimento
2 potatoes
White pepper
1 shallot
grated nutmeg
3 tbsp sunflower oil
Seasoned Salt
750 ml of water
1 teaspoon gluten- and yeast-free vegetable broth without glutamate

PREPARATION:

Wash and peel the potatoes and kohlrabi. Then cut the kohlrabi into pieces. Finely chop the potatoes and shallot. Heat the oil in a saucepan. Sauté the shallots in it. Then add the potatoes and kohlrabi and let everything simmer for another 2 minutes. Deglaze everything with the water and the vegetable stock and bring everything to a boil. Cook the soup for another 15-20 minutes. Then season everything with the spices and puree. Wash and finely chop the parsley and sprinkle over the soup.

KOHLRABI AND CARROT SOUP: INGREDIENTS FOR 4 SERVINGS:

200 g kohlrabi / 400 g carrots
salt and pepper
40 g onions
1 tsp curry
10 g ginger
150 ml coconut milk
1 small chilli pepper
600 ml vegetable stock
20 g butter
Coriander green
some coconut milk

PREPARATION:

Peel the onion and carrots. Roll both dice. Peel and finely chop the ginger. Halve, core and finely chop the chilli pepper. Melt the butter in a saucepan. Steam the chilli, carrots, ginger and onion in it. Deglaze everything with the coconut milk and vegetable stock. Season the whole thing with the spices and simmer for 20 minutes over low heat. In the meantime, wash, peel and dice the kohlrabi. Puree the finished soup and add the kohlrabi cubes. Let everything simmer again for 8 minutes. Garnish the soup with the coriander greens and coconut milk before serving.

STRAWBERRY SALAD: INGREDIENTS FOR 4 SERVINGS:

For the salad:
1 teaspoon red pepper berries
400 g strawberries
12 basil leaves
100 g rocket
For the dressing:
2 tbsp grape seed oil
2 tbsp Balsamico Bianco / 1 pinch of stevia
salt and pepper

PREPARATION:

Wash the strawberries and remove the greens. Then drain and cut into slices. Wash the rocket too and remove the stalks. Spread both together with the basil on plates. Mix all ingredients for the dressing together and pour over the salad. Garnish with the pepper berries.

LAMB'S LETTUCE WITH MUSHROOMS: INGREDIENTS:

2 tbsp sunflower seeds
300 g lamb's lettuce
1 teaspoon sesame oil
200 g white mushrooms
1 apple
1 avocado
300 g cherry tomatoes
For the dressing:
salt and pepper
1/2 bunch of parsley
4 tbsp olive oil
Juice of half a lemon
1 tbsp agave syrup
2 tbsp apple juice

PREPARATION:

Wash the lamb's lettuce and spin dry. Slice the mushrooms and pit the avocado. Then peel the avocado and cut into strips. Wash the apple and remove the core. Then dice the apple. Finely chop the parsley and mix with the remaining ingredients for the dressing. Heat oil in a pan and briefly toast the sunflower seeds. Mix the lamb's lettuce, mushrooms, tomatoes and apple with the dressing. Scatter the sunflower seeds on top.

FRUITY SALAD: INGREDIENTS FOR 2 SERVINGS:

Lemon juice
100 g celery
salt and pepper
100 g apples
100 g pineapple
2 tbsp lupine yogurt
20 g of lettuce
6 walnuts

PREPARATION:

First peel the celery and cut into strips. Drizzle them with a little lemon juice. Peel the apple and remove the core. Then grate the apple and drizzle with a little lemon juice. Season the yogurt with salt and pepper. Then fold in the apples along with the celery. Then chop the walnuts and dice the pineapple. Mix both with the salad and serve the whole thing on 2 large lettuce leaves.

PASTA SALAD: INGREDIENTS FOR 2 SERVINGS:

salt and pepper
50 g whole wheat pasta
Herbs
50 g carrots

vinegar
1/2 red pepper
1 medium-sized pickle
6 black olives
1 teaspoon olive oil
2 tbsp lupine yogurt

PREPARATION:

Cook the pasta according to the instructions on the packet and rinse in cold water. Then cut the carrots, peppers and cucumber into cubes. Halve the olives. Make a marinade from the yoghurt, vinegar, olive oil, salt and pepper and let the olives steep in it. Then mix everything together and garnish with the herbs.

SPRING SALAD: INGREDIENTS FOR 2 SERVINGS:

salt and pepper
1 tbsp oregano
2 medium-sized tomatoes
1 tbsp lemon juice
1 bell pepper
1 tbsp balsamic vinegar
1/2 cucumber
1 tbsp olive oil
1 red onion
8 olives
1 chilli pepper

PREPARATION:

Wash and chop the vegetables. Cut the onion into rings. Mix everything together. Make a dressing from the olive oil, vinegar and lemon juice and add the oregano to taste. Pour the dressing over the salad and stir everything well. Finally, season the whole thing again with salt and pepper.

LENTIL CHILLI: INGREDIENTS FOR 4 SERVINGS:

Mexican spice mix as required
2 cups of red lentils
2 cans of chopped tomatoes
Vegetable broth as needed
some oil
1 can of corn
2 tbsp almond butter
3 red peppers
Chili powder
Green beans as needed
Paprika powder
1 onion
Cayenne pepper
2 cloves of garlic
pepper

PREPARATION:

Bring 4 cups of vegetable stock to the boil and let the lentils boil in it for about 10 minutes. In the meantime, fry the whole onion in a saucepan. Cut the peppers into cubes and add to the onion together with the beans. Deglaze the whole thing with the tomatoes and season. Press the garlic and add it too. Then add the corn and finally the cooked lentils. Finally stir in the almond butter and season to taste again.

CARROT AND ALMOND SOUP: INGREDIENTS FOR 2 SERVINGS:

1 heaped teaspoon dried coriander
some oil
1 pinch of salt
1 onion
1 level teaspoon instant vegetable stock
400 g carrots
1 cm of fresh ginger

100 ml almond milk

PREPARATION:

Dice the onion and ginger. Also cut the carrots into cubes. Heat the oil in a pan. Sweat the onion in it. Then add the ginger and fry together with the carrots with the lid closed for a few minutes. Dissolve the vegetable stock in the almond milk and use it to deglaze the carrots. Mix everything together well. Cook the carrots al dente over a low heat. Finally, season everything with the coriander and arrange on a plate.

POTATO SALAD WITH LEMON DRESSING: INGREDIENTS FOR 1 SERVING:

Herbs to taste
400 g waxy potatoes
1 teaspoon of hemp seeds
salt and pepper
1/2 onion
1 tsp grained vegetable broth
2 tbsp olive oil
1/2 lemon

PREPARATION:

Boil the potatoes in their skins and let them cool. Then peel and cut into slices. Mix the vegetable stock in hot water and pour over the potatoes. Squeeze the lemon and mix the lemon juice with the oil and spices. Cut the onion into rings and add to the potatoes together with the hemp seeds. Then spread the dressing over it and mix everything well.

FRIED BROCCOLI: INGREDIENTS FOR 2 SERVINGS:

Salt and cayenne pepper
some rapeseed oil
1 tsp grained vegetable broth

1 red onion
2 heaped teaspoons of chestnut flour
500 g broccoli
150 ml almond milk
400 g mushrooms

PREPARATION:

Separate the florets from the broccoli. Cut the mushrooms into slices and dice the onion. Cook the broccoli, heat the oil in a pan and fry the onion in it. Then add the mushrooms and fry. Season everything with the vegetable stock, salt and cayenne pepper. Deglaze the mushrooms with half of the almond milk and add the finished broccoli. Mix everything well. Mix the chestnut flour with the remaining almond milk until smooth and stir into the vegetables.

BELL PEPPER PAN: INGREDIENTS FOR 1 SERVING:

1 cm ginger
150 g red pointed peppers
1 pinch of salt
150 g green pointed peppers
1 teaspoon coconut flour
150 g white pointed peppers
100 ml creamy coconut milk
1 teaspoon coconut oil
1 clove of garlic
1 onion

PREPARATION:

Wash and core the peppers. Cut the pulp into strips. Halve the onion and also cut into slices. Cut the garlic and ginger into fine cubes. Heat the coconut oil in a pan and steam the onion. Then add the ginger and garlic. Then add the peppers and heat everything for a few minutes while stirring. Deglaze with the coconut milk and reduce the heat. Let cook with the lid closed. Finally, season everything with salt.

POTATO AND VEGETABLE STEW: INGREDIENTS FOR 2 SERVINGS:

2 tsp sambal oelek
some oil
200 ml vegetable broth
1 onion
300 ml almond milk
6 small potatoes
2 large, red pointed peppers
500 g broccoli

PREPARATION:

Divide the broccoli into florets. Peel the potatoes and the onion and cut into cubes. Core and dice the peppers. Heat some oil in a saucepan. Steam the onion in it. Then add the potatoes and fry them. Then add the remaining vegetables. Deglaze everything with the almond milk and vegetable stock. Finally, season the stew with the sambal oelek. Cook the whole thing with the lid closed and low heat until the desired consistency is achieved.

BROCCOLI AND ALMOND PAN: INGREDIENTS FOR 2 SERVINGS:

1 pinch of salt
500 g broccoli
1 handful of sliced almonds
100 ml almond milk

Preparation:

First cut the broccoli into florets. Cover the bottom of a pan with almond milk. Then add the broccoli and almonds. Bring everything to the boil and cook over a low heat until the broccoli is tender. Finally, season the whole thing with salt.

CARROT AND PEPPER PAN WITH COCONUT SAUCE: INGREDIENTS FOR 1 SERVING:

1 pinch of salt
1 tbsp oil
4 teaspoons coriander
1 onion
2 tbsp creamy coconut milk
250 g carrots
1 tbsp lemon juice
150 g light green peppers

PREPARATION:

Peel and dice the onion and carrots. Wash the peppers and remove the seeds. Also cut the pulp into cubes. Heat the oil in a pan. Sauté the onion until translucent. Then add the carrots and put the lid on the pan. As soon as the carrots are al dente, add the peppers to the pan and close the lid again. In the meantime, stir the coconut milk with the lemon juice. Add the lemon and coconut milk mixture to the vegetables and stir. Cook everything with the lid closed until the desired firmness is achieved. Season with the coriander and salt.

BELL PEPPER AND CHICKPEA SALAD: INGREDIENTS FOR 1 SERVING:

1 pinch of rose-hot paprika powder
1 can of chickpeas
1/4 teaspoon garam masala
1 tbsp lemon juice
1/4 teaspoon cumin
1 tbsp neutral oil
1/4 teaspoon salt
1 spring onion
1 pinch of chili powder
1/4 teaspoon turmeric
1 bell pepper

PREPARATION:

First wash and chop the peppers. Clean the spring onions and cut into thin rings. Mix the chickpeas and the juice together with the oil, lemon juice, spring onions and bell pepper. Season the whole thing with the spices. Let the salad steep before serving.

MILK SOUP WITH CORIANDER: INGREDIENTS FOR 1 SERVING:

salt
4 coriander leaves
1 tsp grained vegetable broth
300 ml of plant milk
1 tbsp oil

Preparation:

Wash the coriander leaves well. Heat the oil in a pan. Put on the coriander leaves in it. Deglaze everything with the milk. Season to taste with the vegetable stock and salt and simmer everything over low heat with the lid closed. Always stir. Finally puree the whole thing.

GLASS NOODLES WITH VEGETABLES: INGREDIENTS FOR 2 SERVINGS:

1 handful of cashew nuts
1 onion
1 tbsp coconut oil
1 leek
2 tbsp sweet soy sauce
2 carrots
2 tbsp tamari sauce
1 handful of broccoli florets
50 g glass noodles

PREPARATION:

Cut the onion into small pieces. Heat oil in a pan. Sauté the onions in it. In the meantime, cut the carrots and leek into strips. Soak the glass noodles in hot water. Add the carrots to the onions and sauté. Then add the leek, the tamari sauce and the soy sauce. Then put the broccoli in the pan and cook everything with the lid closed. Cut the glass noodles in the water, drain and add to the vegetables. Mix everything together well.

SIMPLE FRIED POTATOES: INGREDIENTS FOR 2 SERVINGS:

salt
1 leek
350 g potatoes
1 red onion
3 tbsp oil

Preparation:

Peel and dice the potatoes. Split and wash the leek. Then cut the leek into short strips. Chop the onion into small pieces. Heat the oil in a pan. Steam the onions in it. Then add the potatoes and fry while turning. Then add the leek and fry as well. Finally, season the fried potatoes with salt.

SPICY VEGETABLE POT: INGREDIENTS FOR 1 SERVING:

50 ml creamy coconut milk
1 tbsp oil
1 level teaspoon of green curry paste
230 g white radish
230 g carrots

PREPARATION:

Cut the radish and carrots into thin strips. Heat oil in a saucepan. Toast the curry paste in it. Then add the vegetables and fry, turning constantly. Then turn down the heat and seal the pot. Steam the vegetables. Gradually stir in the coconut milk. Bring everything to the boil and serve.

BAKED ZUCCHINI PAN: INGREDIENTS FOR 1 SERVING:

2 tbsp fried onions
2 tbsp liquid coconut oil
50 g cheese substitute
1 zucchini
3 tbsp oat cream
200 g fresh, brown mushrooms
salt and pepper
some leek

PREPARATION:

First wash the zucchini and cut into slices together with the
mushrooms. Cut the leek into rings. Heat the coconut oil in a pan. Fry the
zucchini in it. Then add the mushrooms and fry them too. Then add the
leek and steam. Deglaze the whole thing with the oat cream and
stir. Season everything to taste with the spices. Then fold in the
cheese. Finally, distribute the fried onions on top and mix everything
together.

VEGETABLE ROULADES: INGREDIENTS FOR 2 SERVINGS:

salt and pepper
400 g potatoes
1 pinch of nutmeg
200 g pumpkin
1 pinch of cayenne pepper
1 red pepper
3 tbsp oil
1 zucchini
200 ml vegetable broth
2 cloves of garlic
200 ml vegetable broth
1 can of chunky tomatoes
5 large savoy cabbage leaves

1 onion

PREPARATION:

Let the savoy cabbage leaves cook in boiling salted water for about 4–5 minutes. Then rinse with cold water and roll dry with a rolling pin. Peel and dice the potatoes. Then boil them in salted water and then pour them off. Mash the potatoes and season with nutmeg. Prepare the pumpkin according to the same principle. Then season the pumpkin with cayenne pepper. Dice the onion and sauté in a saucepan with oil. Deglaze these with the tomatoes and add the stock. Let the whole thing boil for a few minutes and then put in a baking dish. Fry the garlic with a little oil and add the peppers. Season everything with salt and pepper. Stuff the savoy cabbage leaves with the potato mixture, pumpkin mixture and diced paprika and roll up. Then place the finished roulades in the baking dish with the open end facing down. Finally, brush everything with a little oil and bake for about 40 minutes at 180–200 ° C.

COLORFUL, HEALTHY PAN: INGREDIENTS FOR 2 SERVINGS:

1 heaped tablespoon of granulated broth
some oil
200 g broccoli
1 onion
220 g potatoes
3 cm ginger
220 g carrots

PREPARATION:

Divide the broccoli into florets. Cut the ginger into sticks and cut the potatoes and carrots into "French fries". Chop the onion into small pieces. Heat the oil in a pan. Steam the onion in it. Then add the ginger and fry. Then add the potatoes and cook everything over medium heat with the lid closed for about 5 minutes. Then add the broccoli florets and stir everything well. Season the whole thing and close the lid again and steam until the vegetables have the desired firmness.

LIGHT POINTED PEPPER SOUP: INGREDIENTS FOR 3 SERVINGS:

500 ml vegetable broth
some oil
1 red onion
4 red pointed peppers
Preparation:
Wash the peppers and remove the seeds. Cut the pulp into small pieces. Cut the onion into small cubes. Heat the oil in a saucepan. Sauté the onions in it. Then add the peppers and let them sweat. Always stir. Deglaze the whole thing with the vegetable stock and let it simmer. Puree everything at the end.

FRIED POTATOES WITH KOHLRABI: INGREDIENTS FOR 2 SERVINGS:

salt and pepper
500 g kohlrabi
some oil
200 g potatoes
100 ml almond milk
2 heaped teaspoons of wild garlic paste

PREPARATION:

Peel and cut the kohlrabi and potatoes. Heat oil in a pan. Fry the kohlrabi in it. Then add the potatoes and fry them. Mix the wild garlic paste with the almond milk and add to the vegetables. Let everything simmer with the lid closed and low heat. Finally, season the whole thing with salt and pepper.

POTATO AND CELERY STEW: INGREDIENTS FOR 4 SERVINGS:

salt and pepper
20 g green spelled
nutmeg
2 onions
Cayenne pepper
4 carrots
lukewarm water
1.5 kg predominantly waxy potatoes
1/2 celeriac
3 thyme stalks
4 bunches of parsley
2 tbsp vegetable oil
4 tbsp vegetable stock powder

PREPARATION:

Peel and dice the onions, carrots, celery and potatoes. Heat oil in a saucepan. Fry the vegetables together with the green spelled. Then add the thyme with a spice bag to the pot. Deglaze with the stock and water. Let it cook until the potatoes are soft. Then remove the thyme. Chop the parsley and season the stew with the remaining herbs.

PUMPKIN SOUP: INGREDIENTS FOR 4 SERVINGS:

salt and pepper
1 heaped tbsp coconut oil
1 heaped teaspoon red curry paste
1 hokkaido pumpkin
200 ml almond milk
3 red peppers
400 ml vegetable broth

PREPARATION:

Wash and core the peppers. Cut the pulp into cubes. Wash the pumpkin too and remove the seeds. Then dice the pumpkin. Heat the coconut oil in a saucepan. Sweat the pumpkin in it. Then add the paprika and deglaze the whole thing with the vegetable stock. Bring everything to the boil and continue to simmer. In the meantime, mix the almond milk with the curry paste. Add the mixture to the soup and cook until the vegetables are soft. Then puree everything and season with salt and pepper.

RAW VEGETABLES WITH BROWN MILLET: INGREDIENTS FOR 2 SERVINGS:

1 pinch of chili powder
250 ml vegan yogurt
12 peppermint leaves
6 heaped teaspoons of ground brown millet
1 tbsp lemon juice
1 carrot
8 dried figs
4 parsnips

PREPARATION:

Mix the brown millet with the yogurt. Peel the carrots, figs and parsnips and cut into sticks. Add both to the yogurt mixture. Chop the peppermint leaves very finely and add them to the vegetables together with the lemon juice. Mix everything together well and season with the chili powder.

DILL SOUP: INGREDIENTS FOR 2 SERVINGS:

Lemon juice
oil
1 bunch of dill
1 onion
3 heaped teaspoons of grained vegetable stock

500 ml of vegetable milk

PREPARATION:

Heat the oil in a pot. Finely dice the onion and sauté in the oil. Mix the milk with the vegetable stock. Wash and finely chop the dill. Deglaze the onion with the milk and add the dill. Mix everything well and bring to the boil briefly. Finally, season the soup with lemon juice.

BEETROOT ON SPINACH: INGREDIENTS FOR 1 SERVING:

1 handful of herbs
200 g pre-cooked beetroot
1 tbsp oil
50 g fresh baby spinach
salt and pepper
1 handful of walnuts
1 shot of crema di balsamic vinegar
1 red onion

PREPARATION:

First cut the beetroot into small pieces. Mix the walnuts with the beetroot juice and the finely chopped beetroot. Preheat the oven to 170 ° C. Cut the onion into thin slices. Grease a baking dish with oil and spread the onion in it. Put the whole thing in the oven for about 10 minutes. In the meantime, wash the spinach and place on a plate. Season with salt and pepper. Put the finished onions on a plate and pour the beetroot-walnut mixture into the baking dish. Drizzle with the crema di balsamic vinegar and sprinkle the onions over the top. Put everything back in the oven for about 20 minutes. Finally, spread the beetroot over the spinach.

MUSHROOM PAN: INGREDIENTS FOR 2 SERVINGS:

4 heaping tablespoons of horseradish

2 tbsp ghee
250 g mushrooms
1 onion
2 potatoes
2 cloves of garlic
350 g carrots

PREPARATION:

Heat the ghee in a pan. Chop the onion and garlic into small pieces. Sauté both in the pan until translucent. Cut the carrots into sticks and dice the potatoes. Wash and slice the mushrooms. Add the carrots to the onions and fry for a few minutes with the lid closed. Then add the potatoes and close the pan again. Then add the mushrooms and fry everything again with the lid closed. Then reduce the heat and steam the vegetables. Finally add the horseradish and stir everything well. Season everything with salt and pepper before serving.

CELERY AND PEPPER PAN: INGREDIENTS FOR 1 SERVING:

1 heaped teaspoon of granulated broth
1 tbsp coconut oil
100 ml of water
300 g celery
1/2 pk. Herbal mixture
2 red pointed peppers

PREPARATION:

Cut the celery into cubes. Core the peppers and also cut into cubes. Heat the oil in a pan. Fry the celery in it. Then add the bell pepper and pour the vegetable stock over it. Let the whole thing fry briefly with the lid closed. Then deglaze with water and let everything cook. Finally season with the herbs and stir.

VEGETABLE PATTIES: INGREDIENTS FOR 2 SERVINGS:

oil
300 g Hokkaido pumpkin
pepper
300 g carrots
2 teaspoons of curry powder
200 g peppers
3 tsp vegetable broth
1 onion
6 teaspoons of flour
2 cloves of garlic

PREPARATION:

Finely grate the pumpkin and carrots. Finely chop the peppers, onions and garlic. Mix all ingredients together. Shape the mixture into small balls and flatten them a little. Fry the patties in a pan with fat.

PUMPKIN STEW: INGREDIENTS FOR 2 SERVINGS:

2 teaspoons ground tiger nuts
oil
200 ml vegetable broth
2 leeks
1/2 hokkaido pumpkin

Preparation:

Cut the leek into rings. Core and dice the pumpkin. Heat the oil in a pot. Fry the leek. Then add the pumpkin and stir everything together. Deglaze with the vegetable stock and let cook. Stir in the tiger nuts before serving.

POTATO SOUP: INGREDIENTS FOR 2 SERVINGS:

1 pinch of nutmeg

2 kohlrabi

oil

2 onions

500 ml vegetable broth

300 g potatoes

Preparation:

Wash the stems and the green leaves of the kohlrabi and cut into small pieces. Heat the oil in a pot. Finely dice the onion and sauté in it. Then add the kohlrabi leaves and stems and fry. Deglaze the whole thing with the vegetable stock. Peel and chop the potatoes. Put these in the pot and bring to the boil briefly. Let everything simmer at a low temperature. As soon as the vegetables are soft, puree the whole thing and season with nutmeg.

CUCUMBER SALAD: INGREDIENTS FOR 1 SERVING:

1/4 cucumber

chives

1 tomato

basil

1/2 green pepper

1 bunch of spring onions

For the marinade:

2-3 tbsp olive oil

1 tbsp wine vinegar

salt and pepper

PREPARATION:

Wash the cucumber and cut into sticks. Cut the tomato into wedges. Core the peppers and cut into sticks. Cut the onions into rings and finely chop the basil and chives. Mix everything together. Mix all ingredients for the marinade and pour over the salad.

POTATO SALAD: INGREDIENTS FOR 4 SERVINGS:

chives
750 g of fat potatoes
1 teaspoon mustard
2 tbsp cider vinegar
salt and pepper
3 tbsp sunflower oil
100 g onions
5 tbsp beef soup

PREPARATION:

Wash the potatoes and put them in cold water with salt. Boil the potatoes in it until soft, then rinse and peel. Cut the potatoes into slices. Chop the onions and mix with the rest of the ingredients. Mix everything with the still warm potatoes and garnish with chives before serving.

SPRING ROLLS: INGREDIENTS FOR 4 PERSONS:

salt and pepper
1 packet of rice paper for spring rolls
olive oil
3 carrots
Chilli flakes
1 cucumber
1 packet of cress
1 package of green asparagus
1 red pepper
For the dip:
3 teaspoons of pink berries
1 pk. Herbal Hollandaise

PREPARATION:

Wash and core the peppers. Cut the pulp into strips. Heat the oil in a pan. Wash the asparagus and cut off the ends. Cook the asparagus in the pan for about 4–6 minutes. Then quench in ice water. Peel the carrots and cut into sticks. Peel the cucumber and remove the seeds. Cut these into strips as well. Mix everything together and serve.

BEETROOT SALAD: INGREDIENTS FOR 2 SERVINGS:

salt and pepper
2 cooked beetroot
Lemon juice
1 lettuce heart
2 stalks of spring onions
4 red tomatoes
1 tbsp chopped parsley
4 yellow tomatoes
1 tbsp nut oil
3 tbsp pomegranate seeds
2 tsp hot mustard
2 tbsp cashew nuts
2 tbsp pomegranate syrup

PREPARATION:

Mix the pomegranate syrup, mustard and oil. Season the vinaigrette with salt, pepper and a little lemon juice. Roughly chop the cashew nuts and toast them in a pan without fat. Wash and dry the lettuce heart. Remove the yellow leaves from the stalk. Wash the tomatoes and spring onions and then cut them into slices. Wash and finely chop the parsley. Cut one of the beetroot into slices and arrange on a plate. Dice the rest of the beetroot and place in the center of the plate. Drape the lettuce heart and tomatoes around. Sprinkle the whole thing with the dressing. Finally sprinkle the parsley, spring onions and cashew nuts on top.

GRAPEFRUIT SALAD: INGREDIENTS FOR 4 PERSONS:

Chilli flakes
1 teaspoon aniseed
salt and pepper
3 red onions
50 ml grapefruit juice
1 bunch of spring onions
10 tbsp olive oil
2 bulbs of fennel with green
1 lime
2 rosé grapefruit

PREPARATION:

For the marinade, roast the anise seeds in a pan without fat. Chop the fennel greens. Fillet the grapefruit while collecting the juice. Squeeze the lime. Mix the olive oil with the grapefruit juice, the lime juice, the fennel green and the aniseed. Season to taste with salt, pepper and chilli flakes. Wash the fennel, remove the inner stalk and slice the fennel into strips. Peel and finely slice the onions. Mix the onions and fennel with the marinade. Wash the spring onions and cut into thin rings. Use the green as well. Arrange the salad and spread the grapefruit wedges over it. Sprinkle the whole thing with the spring onions and let sit in the fridge for 15 minutes.

SPINACH SOUP: INGREDIENTS FOR 2 SERVINGS:

fresh coriander
500 g fresh spinach
peanuts
1 can of coconut milk
salt and pepper
1 onion
Chili powder
1 tbsp peanut butter

some ginger
2 tbsp lemon juice
2 tbsp vegetable stock powder
200 ml almond milk

PREPARATION:

Cut the onion and ginger into small pieces. Fry both in a little coconut oil. Wash the spinach and add it together with the coconut milk, almond milk and vegetable stock powder. Let the whole thing simmer for about 10 minutes. Finally puree everything and season with the lemon juice, salt, pepper, peanut butter and the chili powder. Chop the peanuts and garnish the soup with the peanuts and coriander.

FRIES WITH MAYONNAISE WITH A DIFFERENCE: INGREDIENTS FOR 2 SERVINGS:

salt and pepper
2 celery bulbs
1 teaspoon vegetable stock powder
2 tbsp coconut oil
2 tbsp lemon juice
1 soft avocado
approx. 50 ml almond milk

PREPARATION:

Peel the celery and cut into sticks. Heat the coconut oil in a pan. Fry the celery in it for about 20 minutes. In the meantime, peel and stone the avocado. Puree the pulp with the lemon juice and almond milk. Season the whole thing with the spices and the vegetable stock powder.

CARROT PUDDING: INGREDIENTS FOR 4 SERVINGS:

Pistachios
300 g carrots

2 tbsp rose water
400 ml almond milk
6–8 dates
1 teaspoon Indian spice mix "Garam Masala"
3 tbsp corn starch
1 teaspoon vanilla powder

PREPARATION:

First peel the carrots and cut them into small pieces. Puree 200 ml almond milk with the dates and carrots. Bring the whole thing to the boil in a saucepan with the remaining almond milk, corn starch, spice mixture and vanilla. Season the pudding with the rose water and sprinkle the pistachios over it.

VEGETABLE SPAGHETTI WITH MUSHROOM SAUCE: INGREDIENTS FOR 2 PEOPLE:

salt and pepper
2 sweet potatoes
Chili powder
300 g mushrooms
1 tbsp vegetable stock powder
400 ml almond milk
2 tbsp yeast flakes
1 tbsp coconut oil
2 tbsp almond butter
1 tbsp coconut oil
1 onion

PREPARATION:

Preheat the oven to 170 ° C. Peel the potatoes and use the spiral cutter to make spaghetti. Place these on a baking sheet lined with baking paper and bake the spaghetti for about 25 minutes. In the meantime, cut the onion into small pieces. Heat the coconut oil in a pan and fry the onion in it. Then add the mushrooms, almond milk, almond butter, spices and vegetable stock. Puree the whole thing and heat it over low heat. Finally stir in the yeast flakes.

Potato and pointed cabbage pan with coconut milk

INGREDIENTS FOR 2 SERVINGS:: SALT AND PEPPER

6 potatoes
1 pointed cabbage
150 ml coconut milk
1 bell pepper
1 tsp curry
2 carrots
2 teaspoons of turmeric
2 onions
2 tbsp olive oil

PREPARATION:

Wash the cabbage and remove the stalk. Then cut the cabbage into fine strips. Peel and dice the onions. Peel and dice the potatoes and carrots. Wash the peppers and cut into strips. Heat the oil in a pan. Fry the onions in it. Then add the carrots and potatoes. Fry everything for about 10 minutes. Then add the cabbage and cook for another 3 minutes. Cook the cabbage over low heat. Finally stir in the coconut milk and bring to the boil. Season to taste with the spices and serve.

QUINOA WITH PEANUT SAUCE: INGREDIENTS FOR 2 SERVINGS:

30 g pomegranate seeds
100 g quinoa
50 g baby spinach
1 tsp turmeric powder
1 tbsp peanut kernels
salt and pepper
1 pinch of chilli flakes
1/2 celeriac

1 tbsp peanut butter
1 carrot
100 g lupine yogurt
1 teaspoon olive oil
2 parsley stalks
dried thyme
Paprika powder
dried marjoram

PREPARATION:

Rinse the quinoa and cook for 15 minutes with twice the amount of salted water and turmeric. Then let the quinoa soak. In the meantime, peel and dice the celery and carrots. Heat the oil in a pan. Steam the vegetables in it for about 10 minutes over medium heat. Season the vegetables with the spices, salt and pepper. Wash the parsley and shake dry. Then finely chop the parsley. Mix the peanut butter with the yogurt and half of the parsley. Season the whole thing with salt, pepper and the chilli flakes. Chop the peanuts. Serve the spinach with the quinoa. Spread the vegetables on top and drizzle with the sauce. Garnish with the rest of the parsley, the peanuts and the pomegranate seeds.

VEGETABLE SOUP WITH POTATOES: INGREDIENTS FOR 2 SERVINGS:

1 pinch of cayenne pepper
250 g celery
125 ml coconut milk
200 g potatoes
1/2 teaspoon turmeric powder
1 onion
salt and pepper
1 piece of ginger
2 carrots
2 tbsp coconut oil
500 ml vegetable broth

PREPARATION:

Wash, peel and chop the vegetables, except for the carrots, and the ginger. Approx. Dice 50 g celery. Heat oil in a saucepan. Steam the onion and then the ginger in it. Then add the vegetables and steam them too. Deglaze with the broth and cook over medium heat for about 15 minutes. In the meantime, peel and dice the carrots. Heat 1 tablespoon of oil in a pan. Fry the carrots and the celery cubes for 7 minutes. Season everything with turmeric, salt and pepper. Add the coconut milk to the soup and puree the soup. Season everything with salt, pepper and cayenne pepper. Finally add the diced vegetables and stir.

POTATO AND BRUSSELS SPROUTS PANCAKES: INGREDIENTS FOR 2–3 PEOPLE:

Rock salt
1 kg of Brussels sprouts
600 g potatoes
nutmeg
1 tbsp grated almonds
mace
1 tbsp coconut oil
black pepper
Juice of half a lemon
Smoked salt

PREPARATION:

Clean the Brussels sprouts. Melt the coconut oil in a saucepan. Roast the Brussels sprouts in it with the lid closed. Then add the lemon juice. Deglaze the Brussels sprouts with the smoked salt and 100 ml of water. Cook the Brussels sprouts for about 15 minutes, stirring gently. Then season with pepper, nutmeg and mace to taste. Peel and grate the potatoes. Fold the almonds and salt into the potato mixture. Heat the oil in a pan. Press the potato mixture into the pan. Spread the Brussels sprouts on top and press in gently. Cover the pan with a lid and fry the potato and Brussels sprouts fritters over medium heat. Then turn the pancake and fry from the other side. Finally sprinkle with parsley and serve.

OVEN BAKED VEGETABLES: INGREDIENTS FOR 2 SERVINGS:

some parsley leaves
450 g carrots
1 tbsp sunflower seeds
320 g fennel
2 tbsp olive oil
300 g red onions
1/2 teaspoon pepper
1/2 teaspoon hot paprika powder
1 teaspoon salt
1 tbsp lemon juice
1 tbsp agave syrup
2 tbsp balsamic vinegar

PREPARATION:

First preheat the oven to 220 ° C. Peel the carrots and cut in half lengthways. Peel the onions. Wash the fennel and remove the stem. Then cut the onions and fennel into wedges. Mix the vegetables with 2 tablespoons of olive oil and salt. Spread the vegetables on a baking sheet and cook in the oven for about 30–40 minutes. In the meantime, mix the agave syrup with the lemon juice, balsamic vinegar, pepper and paprika powder. Spread the dressing over the finished vegetables and serve. Sprinkle with the parsley and sunflower seeds.

CHICKPEA AND ZUCCHINI PAN: INGREDIENTS FOR 2 SERVINGS:

salt and pepper
3 zucchini
1 teaspoon of yeast flakes
1 can of chickpeas
1 pinch of cayenne pepper

1 clove of garlic
1-2 tablespoons chopped parsley
1 tbsp olive oil
1-2 tbsp sesame seeds

PREPARATION:

Cut the zucchini into slices. Heat the oil in a pan. Fry the zucchini in it for about 5 minutes. Allow the chickpeas to drain off. Peel the garlic and cut into cubes. Add the garlic with the chickpeas to the zucchini and sauté for another 5 minutes. Finally, season everything with the herbs, sesame seeds and spices.

EGGPLANT CHICKPEAS OUT OF THE OVEN: INGREDIENTS FOR 2 SERVINGS:

2 tbsp pistachios
400 g eggplant
2 tbsp pomegranate
100 g pre-cooked chickpeas
1/4 teaspoon smoked paprika powder
1 red onion
1/4 teaspoon pepper
1 clove of garlic
1/2 teaspoon salt
50 g Swiss chard
1 tbsp lemon juice
1 tsp sambal oelek
1 tbsp agave syrup
1 teaspoon sesame oil
2 tbsp olive oil
For the dressing:
1/4 teaspoon salt
1 tbsp lemon juice
1 tbsp water
1 teaspoon tahini
2 tbsp lupine yogurt

PREPARATION:

First preheat the oven to 180 ° C. In the meantime, cut the eggplant into cubes and the onion into rings. Chop the garlic. Mix the aubergine with the sambal oelek, the olive oil, the lemon juice, the sesame oil, the agave syrup, salt and pepper as well as the paprika powder. Then mix in the onions, garlic and chickpeas. Spread the vegetables on a baking sheet and bake for 20 minutes. Mix all ingredients for the dressing together. Wash the chard and arrange on plates. Spread the vegetables on top and pour the dressing on top. Finally, garnish with the pistachios and pomegranate.

HERBAL POLENTA WITH ASPARAGUS: INGREDIENTS FOR 2 SERVINGS:

Pine nuts

500 g green asparagus

2 tbsp lemon juice

4–6 sage leaves

1 onion

5 stalks of lemon thyme

1 garlic yeast

1 tbsp vegetable margarine

120 g minute polenta

1/2 teaspoon freshly ground nutmeg

500 ml of water

1 tbsp yeast flakes

1/2 teaspoon salt

1 pinch of pepper

PREPARATION:

First wash the asparagus. Cut off the dry ends. Place the asparagus on a baking sheet and season with salt, pepper and lemon juice. Spread 1 tablespoon of oil over it. Bake the asparagus for 12–15 minutes at 180 ° C. In the meantime, finely chop the onion and garlic. Heat 1 tablespoon of oil in a saucepan. Steam the onion and garlic in it. Deglaze everything with water and stir in the polenta. Season everything with nutmeg, yeast flakes, salt and pepper. Let the polenta simmer for 5 minutes. Pluck the thyme from the stalks and cut the sage. Stir the margarine and herbs into the polenta. Mix everything well and let it steep. Arrange the polenta and serve the asparagus on top. Put the pine nuts and a little lemon juice on top.

GRAPE AND VEGETABLE SALAD: INGREDIENTS FOR 2 SERVINGS:

2 tbsp nuts
2 carrots
150 g of grapes
250 g beetroot
60 g spinach
For the vinaigrette:
salt and pepper
2 tbsp lemon juice
6 mint leaves
2 tbsp olive oil
1 teaspoon mustard
1 tbsp agave syrup

PREPARATION:

Peel the carrots and beetroot and cut into strips. Halve the grapes. Mix the beetroot, carrots and grapes with the nuts. Chop the mint and mix with the remaining ingredients for the vinaigrette. Pour the vinaigrette over the salad and sprinkle some nuts over it.

GREEN BOWL WITH FRIED POTATOES: INGREDIENTS FOR 2 SERVINGS:

salt and pepper
500 g small, boiled potatoes
Paprika powder
200 g baby broccoli
Cayenne pepper
1 romaine lettuce

3 tbsp frying oil
1 clove of garlic
1/2 avocado
For the dressing:
cress
40 g cashew nuts
some lemon juice
80 ml of water
salt and pepper
1 1/2 tsp miso paste
Juice of half a lemon
3 tbsp olive oil

PREPARATION:

Soak the cashew nuts for 2 hours. Wash the broccoli. Heat 1 tablespoon of oil in a pan. Cook the broccoli in it for 10–12 minutes until al dente. Cut the garlic and add to the broccoli for the last 5 minutes. Season with salt and pepper. Halve the potatoes and fry in a pan with 1 tablespoon of oil for 10 minutes. Season the potatoes with salt and pepper as well as with paprika powder and a little cayenne pepper. Remove the stalk from the romaine lettuce. Halve the salad and fry for 3–5 minutes. Drain the cashew nuts. Mix and puree all ingredients for the dressing. Pit the avocado and cut into slices. Mix everything and serve.

SAVOY-CURRY PAN WITH COCONUT MILK: INGREDIENTS FOR 2 SERVINGS:

salt and pepper
250 g savoy cabbage
1 tsp green curry paste
1 small zucchini
150 ml creamy coconut milk

PREPARATION:

Clean the savoy cabbage and cut into thin strips. Finely chop the zucchini. Mix the coconut milk with the curry paste in a saucepan and heat. Cook the savoy cabbage and zucchini over medium heat with the lid closed. Finally, season everything with salt and pepper.

WARM SALAD: INGREDIENTS FOR 2 SERVINGS:

salt and pepper
1 kohlrabi
parsley
2 potatoes
olive oil

Preparation:

Clean and dice the kohlrabi. Cook the kohlrabi cubes in a little salted water. In the meantime, peel the potatoes, dice them and cook them. Mix the finished kohlrabi and the finished potatoes. Spread some olive oil over it. Finely chop the parsley and season the warm salad with salt, pepper and parsley.

VEGETABLE JELLIES: INGREDIENTS FOR 4 PERSONS:

1 pinch of herbal salt
2 carrots
1 pinch of black clover
2 spring onions
1 pinch of marjoram
1 clove of garlic
1 tsp agar agar
1/2 red pepper
1 tbsp fresh, chopped herbs
1/2 yellow pepper
500 ml vegetable broth without yeast
2 tbsp peas

PREPARATION:

Cut the carrots into sticks. Slice the spring onions, dice the peppers and press the garlic. Cook all the vegetables except the peas in the vegetable stock. Then stir in agar-agar. Let everything cook for 2 minutes. Then add the peas, spices and herbs. Then fill everything into molds and let the brawn cool.

BAKED CARROTS AND PARSNIPS: INGREDIENTS FOR 4 SERVINGS:

3 sprigs of rosemary
500 g parsnips
Seasoned Salt
300 g carrots
5 tbsp coconut oil
Preparation:

First preheat the oven to 200 ° C. Cut the carrots and parsnips into sticks. Spread both on a baking sheet and season with salt. Halve the rosemary sprigs and distribute between the vegetables. Drizzle everything with a little coconut oil and cook in the oven for 30 minutes.

MANGO SALAD: INGREDIENTS:

Juice of half a lemon
2 mangoes
200 g papaya
Preparation:

Peel the fruit and remove the stones. Dice the pulp. Halve the lemon and squeeze it. Drizzle the fruit cubes with the lemon juice. Mix everything together and let it steep for about half an hour.

COOKED POTATOES: INGREDIENTS FOR 2 SERVINGS:

salt and pepper
550 g potatoes
1 teaspoon marjoram
300 ml vegetable broth
1 pinch of chilli flakes
2 tbsp coconut oil

1 teaspoon paprika powder, noble sweet

PREPARATION:

Peel and dice the potatoes. Heat the coconut oil in a pan. Fry the potatoes in it for 3–5 minutes and season with the spices. Then deglaze with the vegetable stock. Let everything simmer for about 15 minutes over medium heat. Stir again and again. Finally, season the potatoes again and serve.

Spaghetti with tomato sauce is a little different

INGREDIENTS FOR 2 SERVINGS:: SPICES

2 zucchini
Hemp cream
4 carrots
garlic
3 tomatoes
Vegetable oil
Onions

Preparation:

Cut the carrots into spaghetti with a spiral cutter. Boil these in a little salted water. In the meantime, dice the onions and garlic cloves. Heat the oil in a pan. Sauté the garlic and onions in it. Dice the tomatoes and add to the onions. Season everything with the spices. Deglaze the tomatoes with the cream. Drain the carrot spaghetti and mix into the sauce.

VEGETABLE STICKS: INGREDIENTS:

Vegetable oil
Parsnips
rosemary
Carrots
Onions
paprika

Preparation:

Wash the vegetables. Peel the parsnips and carrots. Core the peppers. Cut the vegetables into sticks. Dice the onions. Mix the rosemary with the vegetable oil and the onions. Then fold in the vegetables. Spread everything on a baking sheet and bake at 180 ° C until the vegetable sticks are lightly brown.

BEANS WITH SESAME SEEDS: INGREDIENTS FOR 4 SERVINGS:

salt and pepper
600 g French beans
olive oil
3 spring onions
Juice and zest of half a lemon
1/2 chilli pepper
2 tbsp sesame oil
2 tbsp sesame seeds

PREPARATION:

Chop the beans and cook in salted water for 10 minutes. Cut the spring onions into rings. Core the chilli pepper and cut into rings. Heat the sesame oil in a pan. Steam the spring onions and the chilli pepper for 5 minutes while turning. Then stir in the lemon juice and lemon zest. Add the finished beans and season everything with salt and pepper. Steam for 10 minutes. Toast the sesame seeds in a pan. Arrange the beans on a plate and sprinkle the sesame seeds on top.

BRUSSELS SPROUTS WITH ALMONDS: INGREDIENTS FOR 4 SERVINGS:

salt and pepper
700 g Brussels sprouts
2 tbsp spelled breadcrumbs
100 g of chopped almonds
50 g butter
1 clove of garlic
Zest of a lemon

PREPARATION:

First clean the Brussels sprouts and cut off the bottom. Cook the Brussels sprouts in salted water for 5–7 minutes. Then keep the cabbage warm. Heat half of the butter in a pan. Roast the almonds and halved garlic in it. Season the garlic with salt, pepper and lemon zest. Then remove the garlic and put everything aside. Heat the rest of the butter in a saucepan. Toast the breadcrumbs in it. Add the breadcrumbs to the almond mixture. Serve the Brussels sprouts and spread the almond and breadcrumb mixture over them.

POTATO AND KALE STEW: INGREDIENTS FOR 2 SERVINGS:

salt and pepper
250 g kale
ground thyme
250 g potatoes
2 tbsp coconut oil
2 tomatoes
500 ml vegetable stock (without yeast)
2 onions
2 cloves of garlic

PREPARATION:

Clean the cabbage and cut into strips. Cut the potatoes into cubes. Peel the tomatoes and dice the pulp. Finely chop the onions and garlic. Heat coconut oil in a saucepan. Steam the onions and garlic in it. Then add the potatoes and cook for 2 minutes. Deglaze everything with the vegetable stock and season with salt. Simmer for 10 minutes with the lid closed. Then add the kale and cook for 15 minutes. Then add the tomatoes and cook for 3 minutes. Finally season everything with pepper, salt and thyme.

BEAN PAN: INGREDIENTS FOR 4 SERVINGS:

salt and pepper
700 g potatoes
3 tbsp olive oil
500 g green beans
2 sprigs of savory
2 onions
2 sprigs of thyme

PREPARATION:

Wash the potatoes and cook in salted boiling water for 20 minutes. In the meantime, wash the beans and cut them into small pieces. Blanch these in boiling salted water for 8 minutes. Peel the onions and cut into rings. Wash the herbs and gently shake dry. Rinse the finished beans in cold water and let them drain. Drain the potatoes and let them cool. Then peel the potatoes and cut them into slices. Heat 2 tablespoons of oil in a pan and fry the potatoes in it. Season the potatoes with salt and pepper. Heat the remaining oil in a separate pan. Fry the beans, onions, thyme and savory for 8–10 minutes. Then fold everything under the potatoes and season to taste again.

SPICY POTATOES: INGREDIENTS FOR 2 SERVINGS:

Crystal salt
550 g small potatoes
1 teaspoon marjoram
2 tbsp coconut oil
1 pinch of chilli flakes
300 ml vegetable broth
1 teaspoon paprika, noble sweet

PREPARATION:

Wash, peel and dice the potatoes. Heat the oil in a pan. Fry the potatoes in it for 3–5 minutes. Season to taste with the spices. Then deglaze the potatoes with the vegetable stock. Let everything cook for about 15 minutes and stir occasionally.

FRUITY KOHLRABI SALAD: INGREDIENTS FOR 2 SERVINGS:

1 handful of chopped parsley
1 large kohlrabi
1-2 tbsp lemon juice
1 apple
2 tbsp olive oil
2 parsnips
6 tbsp oat cream
1 small piece of ginger

PREPARATION:

Peel and roughly grate the kohlrabi and parsnips. Roughly grate the apple and drizzle with the lemon juice. Finely grate the ginger. Mix all ingredients together. Let the salad stand for 15 minutes. Then season again to taste and serve.

SPRING-LIKE, COLORFUL SALAD: INGREDIENTS FOR 4 SERVINGS:

2 carrots
1 bunch of dandelions
1/2 stick of leek
1 bunch of rocket
1/2 bunch of wild garlic
1 bunch of radishes with leaves
1/2 bunch Postelein

PREPARATION:

Wash and drain the radish leaves, dandelions, wild garlic, rocket and Postelein. Cut everything into small pieces. Wash the radishes and cut into thin slices. Wash the leek and cut into rings. Peel the carrots and cut into chips. Mix everything together.

CAULIFLOWER PAN: INGREDIENTS FOR 2 SERVINGS:

1/2 teaspoon cumin
1 small cauliflower
1/2 teaspoon ginger powder
150 g mustard sprouts
1/2 teaspoon turmeric
2 cloves of garlic
100 ml coconut milk
1 onion
2 tbsp coconut oil
1 bunch of parsley
125 ml vegetable broth without yeast

PREPARATION:

Separate the florets from the cauliflower. Chop the onion and garlic. Heat the coconut oil in a pan and sauté the onion and garlic. Then add the cauliflower. Deglaze everything with the vegetable stock and bring to the boil. Close the pan with a lid and simmer the cauliflower for 5 minutes over medium heat. Then add the sprouts, turmeric, ginger, salt, cumin, pepper and coconut milk. Let everything thicken while stirring constantly. Chop the parsley and pour over the cauliflower.

DESSERTS: APPLE DESSERT

Ingredients for 4 persons:
cinnamon

2 ripe quinces
ground vanilla
250 ml of water
200 g whippable soy cream
80 g stevia
1 teaspoon honey
2 tbsp lemon juice
2 apples

PREPARATION:

First the quinces are rubbed vigorously with a cloth. Then they are peeled, quartered and cut into cubes. The water is boiled with the stevia and lemon juice. Reduce the stevia-lemon water a little and then add the quince cubes. These should cook in the water. The apples are roughly grated and mixed with the honey and lemon juice. Then the apples are seasoned with vanilla and cinnamon. The soy cream is whipped until stiff and half of the cream is folded into the apple mixture. Now the apple cream is divided between 4 glass plates. The quince cubes are drained and added to the apple cream. The rest of the cream is poured over it to decorate.

FRUITY DREAM: INGREDIENTS FOR 2 PEOPLE:

250 g of grapes
2 teaspoons of cornstarch
1 ripe banana
100 ml red fruit juice
2 tsp stevia
150 g fresh or frozen raspberries

PREPARATION:

The cornstarch is stirred with 2 tablespoons of red fruit juice until smooth. The remaining fruit juice is put in a saucepan with the raspberries and brought to the boil. Then the whole thing is simmered for 4–5 minutes on low heat. The mixed cornstarch is now added to the berries and boiled while stirring. Now the stevia is stirred in. Let the berries simmer for about 1 minute and then pour them through a sieve. Strain the berries through the sieve. The bananas are peeled and cut into small cubes. These are mixed into the berry sauce. Finally, the grapes are washed and plucked from the stems and set aside to drain. Then the banana and berry sauce is spread over two dessert plates. The grapes are served on the dessert.

CINNAMON CREAM WITH APPLES: INGREDIENTS FOR 10 PEOPLE:

some lemon balm leaves
1 kg of apples
Juice of one lemon
100 g raisins
250 g whippable soy cream
100 ml apple juice
1/2 teaspoon ground cinnamon
80 g stevia
250 g natural yogurt

PREPARATION:

First the apples are peeled and cored. Then they are quartered and cut into thin slices. The apple slices are placed in a saucepan. Together with the raisins, apple juice, lemon juice and stevia, the apple slices are cooked in the pan for about 5 minutes. The apples should be firm to the bite. Then take the pot off the stove and let it cool down. In the meantime, stir the yogurt with the cinnamon. The cream is whipped until stiff and folded into the yoghurt cream. The cooled apple pieces are distributed on dessert bowls. The cinnamon cream is given over it. For serving, the dessert can be garnished with lemon balm.

BLUEBERRY MUFFINS: INGREDIENTS FOR 12 PIECES:

12 paper muffin cases

200 g whole wheat flour
2 tbsp water
60 g of oatmeal
300 g of oat cream
2 teaspoons of baking soda
180 g stevia
1/2 teaspoon baking soda
2 eggs
250 g blueberries

PREPARATION:

The oven is preheated to 160 ° C. The muffin tin is laid out with the baking molds. Now the flour is mixed with the oat flakes, baking soda and baking powder. The blueberries are cleaned and washed. Then the eggs are whisked and mixed with the stevia, water and oat cream. Now the flour mixture is folded in. Finally, add the blueberries. Pour the finished dough into the muffin molds and bake in the preheated oven for 20-25 minutes. As soon as the baking time is up, take the muffins out of the oven and let them rest for 5 minutes.
Tip: The muffins can also be frozen.

STUFFED COCONUT FIGS: INGREDIENTS FOR 10 PIECES:

10 whole pecans
10 dried figs
10 teaspoons of raw almond butter
1/4 cup fresh desiccated coconut
Preparation:
First the figs are cut lengthways and filled with the almond butter. The filled figs are rolled out in the desiccated coconut and decorated with a pecan nut.

MACADAMIA AND ALMOND CREAM: INGREDIENTS:

1 kg of fresh cherries

300 g macadamia nuts
1/2 teaspoon stevia (more or less depending on your taste)
60 g almonds
1 tbsp vanilla powder
2 cups of fresh almond milk

PREPARATION:

The macadamia nuts and almonds are soaked in water for at least 12 hours. The soaked nuts are now put in a blender. Stevia, almond milk and vanilla powder are added and mixed together until a creamy consistency is obtained. If the consistency is too firm, some almond milk can be added. Now the cream has to rest in the refrigerator for at least 3 hours. The finished cream is served with the cherries.

ESPRESSO COCOA DELICACY: INGREDIENTS FOR 2 SERVINGS:

1 banana
200 ml of sweet whey
50 ml espresso
1 pinch of cocoa
2 teaspoons of cocoa
1 pk. vanilla sugar

PREPARATION:: PREPARE ESPRESSO AND LET IT COOL DOWN.

Then bananas, whey, vanilla sugar and cocoa are combined and mashed. Stir in the espresso and serve with a drinking straw.

COCONUT COOKIES: INGREDIENTS FOR 10 COOKIES:

150 g coconut flakes
2 ripe bananas
Preparation:
Mash the bananas, add the coconut flakes and stir together. Preheat the

oven to 150 ° C. Shape the mixture into cookies and spread them on a baking sheet lined with baking paper. Bake the cookies for 15–20 minutes.

COCONUT CHEESECAKE: INGREDIENTS FOR AN 18 CM SPRINGFORM PAN:

For the ground:
cinnamon
1 banana
6 tbsp ground tiger nuts
For the crowd:
2 bananas
200 g Creamed Coconut

PREPARATION:

First preheat the oven to 170 ° C. Mash the banana for the bottom. Mix in the tiger nuts and some cinnamon. Line the springform pan with baking paper. Spread the banana mixture on the bottom of the springform pan. Bake the finished base for 20-25 minutes. Then let the base cool down. Now set the oven to 100 ° C. Let the creamed coconut soften in a container in the oven. Puree the mixture with the bananas in a blender. Spread the mixture on the cake base and let it harden in the refrigerator.

CARROT CAKE: INGREDIENTS FOR A CAKE: (BAKING PAN 20 X 20 CM)

For the cake:
2 tbsp coconut oil
3 carrots
1/2 teaspoon cinnamon
2 bananas
170 g desiccated coconut
140 g ground almonds
For the topping:
1/2 tbsp coconut oil
150 g white almond butter

25 ml of water
25 ml lime juice

PREPARATION:

Puree the bananas and carrots. Heat the coconut oil in a saucepan. Mix the banana mixture with the almonds, desiccated coconut, cinnamon and coconut oil. Put everything in the baking pan. Mix the almond butter with the water, the lime juice and the liquid coconut oil. Spread the whole thing on the cake. Let the finished cake set in the refrigerator for at least 1 hour.

FRUIT ICE CREAM: INGREDIENTS FOR 4 SERVINGS:

1 tbsp almond butter
1 avocado
100 ml orange juice
1 mango
1 banana

Preparation:

Core the avocado. Remove the pulp and cut into small pieces. Peel the mango and the banana and cut them into small pieces. Freeze everything for a few hours. Let the frozen fruits thaw and mix together with the orange juice and almond butter until creamy.

CUP APPLE PIE: INGREDIENTS FOR 1 CAKE:

1/2 cup raisins
1 cup of ground walnuts
1/2 cup desiccated coconut
1 cup of dates
1/2 cup of fresh apple juice
1/2 cup of raw sunflower seeds
2 1/2 teaspoons of cinnamon
4 cups of grated apples

PREPARATION:

Soak the dates and sunflower seeds in alkaline water, the dates for 15 minutes and the sunflower seeds for 20 minutes. Mix 2/3 of the coconut flakes with the drained dates, sunflower seeds and walnuts. Put the mixture in a cake tin. Mix the grated apples with the cinnamon, apple juice and raisins. Put the apple mixture on the cake base and sprinkle the remaining desiccated coconut on top.

HEARTY GRANOLA BARS: INGREDIENTS FOR 10 BARS:

1/4 teaspoon chili powder
500 g sunflower seeds
1/2 tsp organic coriander powder
1 red pepper
1 teaspoon sea salt
2 celery stalks
2 heaped teaspoons of organic paprika powder
1/2 onion
1 bunch of parsley
1 handful of young spinach leaves
1 teaspoon of minced garlic

PREPARATION:

Soak the sunflower seeds in 120 ml of water overnight. Wash, core and cut the bell peppers. Chop the celery, onion, spinach and parsley as well. Chop the vegetables in a blender. Then add the sunflower seeds and mix again. Shape the mixture into bars and bake in the oven on low heat.

DATE PRALINES: INGREDIENTS FOR 24 PRALINES:

100 g unsweetened desiccated coconut
2 cups of fresh dates
80 ml of water

Preparation:

Bring the dates to the boil with the water and stir occasionally until a paste is formed. Let the mixture cool down and shape into balls. Roll these in the coconut flakes and let them cool in the refrigerator.

DATE SMOOTHIE: INGREDIENTS:

fresh cinnamon
2 fresh dates
1 cup of fresh, chilled coconut milk

Preparation:

Puree the coconut milk with the dates and cinnamon in a blender.

ALMOND AND COCONUT WEDGES: INGREDIENTS:

Juice of half a lemon
200 ml of liquid coconut oil
200 g fresh coconut flakes
220 g of chopped almonds

PREPARATION:

Soak the almonds in water overnight. Then mix all ingredients except for 50 g desiccated coconut. Put the mixture in a baking dish. Sprinkle the remaining desiccated coconut on top. Let everything cool in the refrigerator for about 1 hour. Then cut small pieces out of the mass.

STRAWBERRY PUDDING: INGREDIENTS FOR 2 SERVINGS:

some chopped pistachios
2 tbsp chia seeds
180 g strawberries
100 ml of plant milk
2 tsp stevia
1 teaspoon lemon juice

PREPARATION:

Mix the milk with the chia seeds, lemon juice and 1 teaspoon stevia. Let it soak for at least 2 hours. Stir several times. Put 4–5 strawberries aside. Puree the remaining strawberries with 1 teaspoon stevia. Halve the remaining strawberries and chop the pistachios. Stir the swollen chia seeds once more and layer them in glasses with the strawberry puree. Place the halved strawberries on top.

APPLE-CREAM: INGREDIENTS FOR 2 SERVINGS:

250 g lupine yogurt
360 g apple pulp
1 tbsp lemon juice
4 heaped teaspoons of ground brown millet
1 teaspoon cinnamon
2 heaped tbsp tiger nuts flakes

PREPARATION:: MIX ALL INGREDIENTS AND STIR WELL.

Avocado Mousse
Ingredients for 4 persons:
1 1/2 teaspoons of sea salt
2 avocados
5 dates
200 ml coconut water
2 tbsp raw cocoa
1 tbsp vanilla

PREPARATION:

Stone the avocados and remove the pulp. Mix the pulp with the remaining ingredients. Let the mass solidify in the refrigerator for 4 hours.

STRAWBERRY AND AVOCADO CREAM: INGREDIENTS FOR 2 SERVINGS:

2 ripe avocados
250 g ripe strawberries
1 tbsp agave syrup
2 tbsp coconut oil
For the decoration:
Strawberries
Coconut flakes
Mint leaves

PREPARATION:

Stone the avocados and remove the pulp. Cut the pulp into slices. Wash the strawberries and mix together with the avocado, coconut oil and agave syrup. Pour the cream into bowls and garnish with some strawberries, the mint leaves and the coconut flakes.

FRUIT SALAD: INGREDIENTS:

1/2 tbsp honey
1 banana
15 g of donated almonds
1 orange
25 raisins
Juice of one lemon
1 peach (alternatively nectarine or apricot)
1 pear
1/4 pineapple
1 apple

PREPARATION:

Core the pear, apple and peach and cut into pieces. Peel the pineapple and orange and cut into pieces. Mix everything together. Cut the bananas into slices and drizzle some lemon juice over them. Carefully fold the banana with the almonds and raisins into the salad. Season the whole thing with honey. Let the finished salad stand in the refrigerator for at least 1 hour.

FRUIT SALAD: INGREDIENTS:

1/2 tbsp honey
1 banana
15 g of donated almonds
1 orange
25 raisins
Juice of one lemon
1 peach (alternatively nectarine or apricot)
1 pear
1/4 pineapple
1 apple

PREPARATION:

Core the pear, apple and peach and cut into pieces. Peel the pineapple and orange and cut into pieces. Mix everything together. Cut the bananas into slices and drizzle some lemon juice over them. Carefully fold the banana with the almonds and raisins into the salad. Season the whole thing with honey. Let the finished salad stand in the refrigerator for at least 1 hour.

THE COMPLETE ANTI-INFLAMMATORY FOOD LIST

Beverages

Potential Pro-Inflammatory Ingredients (Avoid/Minimize)

Soft drinks, sweetened (with sugar or artificial sweetener) ‖ Soda, regular ‖ Soda, diet ‖ Milk, dairy ‖ Liquor, hard ‖ Liqueurs ‖ Juice, sweetened ‖ Energy drinks ‖ Beer ‖ Artificially or sugar sweetened drinks

Ingredients That Reduce Inflammation (Eat These)

Wine (limit 4 oz.) ‖ Kombucha ‖ Coffee ‖ Chai (with nondairy milk and no sugar)

Potent Anti-Inflammatory Foods (Eat A Lot)

Water ‖ Tea (Particularly Green Tea)

Condiments
Potential Pro-Inflammatory Ingredients (Avoid/Minimize)
Vinaigrette (store-bought) ‖ Teriyaki sauce (store-bought) ‖ Salsa, with sugar ‖ Salad dressing ‖ Mayonnaise (store-bought) ‖ Ketchup ‖ Cocktail sauce ‖ Barbecue sauce

Ingredients That Reduce Inflammation (Eat These)
Worcestershire sauce ‖ Wasabi ‖ Vinegar, all kinds ‖ Vinaigrette (homemade) ‖ Tomato paste ‖ Teriyaki sauce, sugar-free (homemade) ‖ Tamari ‖ Tahini ‖ Soy sauce ‖ Salsa, sugar-free ‖ Mustard, ground ‖ Mustard, Dijon ‖ Miso ‖ Mayonnaise (homemade) ‖ Hot sauce, sugar-free ‖ Horseradish, prepared, sugar-free ‖ Fish sauce, sugar-free ‖ Anchovy paste

Dairy And Dairy Alternatives
Potential Pro-Inflammatory Ingredients (Avoid/Minimize)
Whipped cream ‖ Sour cream ‖ Nondairy creamer ‖ Kefir, cow's milk ‖ Ice cream ‖ Heavy (whipping) cream ‖ Half-and-half ‖ Goat's milk ‖ Cow's milk (all types) ‖ Cheese, dairy (all types)

Ingredients That Reduce Inflammation (Eat These)
Yogurt, Greek ‖ Yogurt, dairy ‖ Yogurt, coconut, plain, unsweetened ‖ Yogurt, almond, plain, unsweetened ‖ Soymilk, unsweetened ‖ Kefir, water ‖ Hemp milk, unsweetened ‖ Coconut milk, lite, unsweetened ‖ Coconut milk, full-fat, unsweetened ‖ Almond milk, unsweetened

Fats And Oils
Potential Pro-Inflammatory Ingredients (Avoid/Minimize)
Vegetable oil ‖ Sunflower oil ‖ Soybean oil ‖ Shortening ‖ Sesame oil ‖ Safflower oil ‖ Peanut oil ‖ Palm oil ‖ Margarine ‖ Lite olive oil ‖ Hydrogenated oils ‖ Corn oil ‖ Canola oil ‖ Butter

Ingredients That Reduce Inflammation (Eat These)
Macadamia oil ‖ Coconut oil ‖ Avocado oil

Potent Anti-Inflammatory Foods (Eat A Lot)
Extra-Virgin Olive Oil

Fruits
Potential Pro-Inflammatory Ingredients (Avoid/Minimize)
Processed juices with added sugar ‖ Canned fruit in syrup

Ingredients That Reduce Inflammation (Eat These)
Yuzu ‖ Watermelon ‖ Ugli fruit ‖ Tayberry ‖ Tangerine ‖ Tamarind ‖ Strawberry ‖ Star fruit ‖ Satsuma ‖ Santa Claus melon ‖ Salmonberry ‖ Red currant ‖ Raspberry ‖ Raisin ‖ Quince ‖ Prunes ‖ Prickly pear ‖ Pomelo ‖ Pomegranate ‖ Pluot ‖ Plum ‖ Plantain ‖ Pineapple ‖ Persimmon

‖ Persian melon ‖ Pear ‖ Peach ‖ Passionfruit ‖ Papaya ‖ Orange ‖ Olives ‖ Nectarine ‖ Mulberry ‖ Marionberry ‖ Mangosteen ‖ Mango ‖ Mandarin ‖ Lychee ‖ Lime ‖ Lemon ‖ Kumquat ‖ Kiwi ‖ Jackfruit ‖ Huckleberry ‖ Horned melon ‖ Honeydew ‖ Guava ‖ Grapefruit ‖ Grape ‖ Gooseberry ‖ Goji berry ‖ Galia (melon) ‖ Fig ‖ Elderberry ‖ Durian ‖ Dragon fruit ‖ Date ‖ Currant ‖ Cranberry ‖ Coconut ‖ Clementine ‖ Chokecherry ‖ Cherry ‖ Charentais (melon) ‖ Casaba melon ‖ Cantaloupe ‖ Canary melon ‖ Breadfruit ‖ Boysenberry ‖ Blood orange ‖ Blackcurrant ‖ Blackberry ‖ Banana ‖ Avocado ‖ Asian pear ‖ Apricot ‖ Apple ‖ Acai

Potent Anti-Inflammatory Foods (Eat A Lot)
Blueberries

Grains And Starches
Ingredients That May
Trigger Inflammation (Avoid/Minimize)
Wheat, refined ‖ Rice, white ‖ Potato starch ‖ Pasta ‖ Oatmeal, instant, with sugar ‖ Flour, white ‖ Cereal ‖ Bread, white ‖ Baked goods (bread, cookies, donuts, pies, etc.)

Ingredients That Reduce Inflammation (Eat These)
Wild rice ‖ Wheat, whole ‖ Wheat, cracked ‖ Teff ‖ Rye ‖ Rice, brown ‖ Quinoa ‖ Oats, rolled ‖ Millet ‖ Kamut ‖ Farro ‖ Cornstarch ‖ Corn ‖ Bulgur ‖ Buckwheat ‖ Barley ‖ Arrowroot ‖ Amaranth

Meats, Poultry, Fish, And Proteins
Potential Pro-Inflammatory Ingredients (Avoid/Minimize)
Whey protein ‖ Trout, fried ‖ Shrimp, fried ‖ Scallops, fried ‖ Sausage ‖ Salami ‖ Pork, ground ‖ Liver (all types) ‖ Lamb, rib chops ‖ Lamb, rack ‖ Kidney (all types) ‖ Hot dogs ‖ Heart (all types) ‖ Ham ‖ Gizzards ‖ Foie gras ‖ Fish, fried ‖ Farmed seafood ‖ Deli meats ‖ Cured meats ‖ Chicken, fried ‖ Catfish, fried ‖ Brains (all types) ‖ Bologna ‖ Beef, rib eye ‖ Beef, prime rib ‖ Beef, New York strip ‖ Beef, feedlot ‖ Bacon

Ingredients That Reduce Inflammation (Eat These)
Venison ‖ Turkey, free-range, skinless ‖ Tilapia, wild-caught ‖ Sturgeon, wild-caught ‖ Snapper ‖ Skate ‖ Shrimp ‖ Scallops ‖ Razor clams ‖ Pork, top loin roast ‖ Pork, tenderloin (preferably pastured) ‖ Pork, sirloin roast ‖ Pork, rib chop ‖ Pork, center loin chop ‖ Pork, boneless top loin chop ‖ Orange roughy ‖ Mussels ‖ Lamb, very lean cuts ‖ Halibut ‖ Elk ‖ Eggs ‖ Duck, free-range, skinless ‖ Cod ‖ Clams ‖ Chicken, free-range, skinless ‖ Catfish, wild-caught ‖ Bison, lean ‖ Beef, lean or very lean ‖ Bass, wild-caught ‖ Anchovy

Potent Anti-Inflammatory Foods (Eat A Lot)

Salmon (and other fatty fish including tuna, mackerel, sardines, and trout)

Nuts, Seeds, And Legumes
Ingredients That Reduce Inflammation (Eat These)

Walnuts, raw ‖ Sunflower seeds ‖ Soybeans ‖ Sesame seeds ‖ Poppy seeds ‖ Pistachios, raw ‖ Pinto beans ‖ Pine nuts ‖ Pecans, raw ‖ Peas, sugar snap ‖ Peas, split ‖ Peas, snow ‖ Peas, green ‖ Peas, black-eyed ‖ Peanuts, raw ‖ Peanut butter ‖ Macadamia nuts, raw ‖ Lima beans ‖ Lentils ‖ Kidney beans ‖ Hazelnuts, raw ‖ Flaxseed ‖ Fava beans ‖ Cocoa beans (dark chocolate, cocoa powder) ‖ Chickpeas (garbanzo beans) ‖ Chia seeds ‖ Cashews, raw ‖ Brazil nuts, raw ‖ Black beans ‖ Almonds, raw ‖ Almond butter ‖ Adzuki beans

Potent Anti-Inflammatory Foods (Eat A Lot)

NUTS

Sweeteners
Potential Pro-Inflammatory Ingredients (Avoid/Minimize)

Xylitol ‖ Syrup, brown rice, corn, high fructose corn, maple (artificial), simple ‖ Sugar, brown and powdered ‖ Sugar alcohols ‖ Sucralose (Splenda) ‖ Sorbitol ‖ Saccharine ‖ Molasses, refined ‖ Mannitol ‖ Erythritol ‖ Aspartame (NutraSweet) ‖ Agave nectar ‖ Acesulfame-K (Acesulfame potassium)

Ingredients That Reduce Inflammation (Eat These)

Stevia ‖ Maple syrup, pure ‖ Honey

Vegetables
Potential Pro-Inflammatory Ingredients (Avoid/Minimize)

Zucchini ‖ Yam ‖ Watercress ‖ Water chestnut ‖ Wakame ‖ Turnip greens ‖ Turnip ‖ Tomatoes, canned (sugar-free) ‖ Tomato sauce (sugar-free) ‖ Tomatillo ‖ Swiss chard ‖ Sweet potato ‖ Sunchoke ‖ Sprouts ‖ Spinach ‖ Spaghetti squash ‖ Shallots ‖ Scallions ‖ Rutabaga ‖ Rapini ‖ Purslane ‖ Pumpkin ‖ Potatoes ‖ Pea pods ‖ Pattypan squash ‖ Parsnip ‖ Onions ‖ Okra ‖ Nori ‖ Nopales ‖ Mustard greens ‖ Mushrooms ‖ Lettuce (all types) ‖ Kohlrabi Leeks ‖ Jicama

Ingredients That Reduce Inflammation (Eat These)

Hearts of palm ‖ Grape leaves ‖ Frisée ‖ Fennel ‖ Endive ‖ Eggplant ‖ Edamame ‖ Dulse ‖ Cucumber ‖ Corn ‖ Collard greens ‖ Chayote ‖ Celery ‖ Celeriac (celery root) ‖ Cauliflower ‖ Carrots ‖ Cabbage ‖ Butternut squash ‖ Brussels sprouts ‖ Broccolini ‖ Broccoli rabe ‖ Bok choy ‖ Beets ‖ Beet greens ‖ Beans, green ‖ Asparagus ‖ Arugula ‖ Artichoke ‖ Acorn squash

Potent Anti-Inflammatory Foods (Eat A Lot)

Tomatoes ‖ spinach ‖ kale ‖ broccoli ‖ bell peppers

Herbs, And Spices

Potential Pro-Inflammatory Ingredients (Avoid/Minimize)

Table salt ‖ Spice blends with sugar ‖ Seasoning salt ‖ Garlic salt

Ingredients That Reduce Inflammation (Eat These)

Vanilla bean ‖ Thyme ‖ Tarragon ‖ Sumac ‖ Spearmint ‖ Salt, Himalayan pink and sea ‖ Sage ‖ Saffron ‖ Rhubarb ‖ Red pepper flakes ‖ Radish ‖ Radicchio ‖ Pepper (black) ‖ Parsley ‖ Paprika ‖ Oregano ‖ Orange zest ‖ Onion powder ‖ Nutmeg ‖ Mustard seed ‖ Mustard powder ‖ Mint ‖ Marjoram ‖ Mace ‖ Lime zest ‖ Lemongrass ‖ Lemon zest ‖ Lemon pepper ‖ Lavender ‖ Juniper berry ‖ Horseradish ‖ Herbes de Provence ‖ Garam masala ‖ Galangal ‖ Fenugreek ‖ Fennel seed ‖ Dill ‖ Curry powder ‖ Cumin ‖ Coriander ‖ Cilantro ‖ Chives ‖ Chipotle ‖ Chinese five-spice powder ‖ Chile peppers ‖ Chamomile ‖ Celery salt ‖ Cayenne ‖ Cassia ‖ Caraway ‖ Bay leaves ‖ Basil ‖ Asafoetida ‖ Anise, star ‖ Anise ‖ Allspice

Potent Anti-Inflammatory Foods (Eat A Lot)

TURMERIC ‖ ROSEMARY ‖ GINGER ‖ GARLIC ‖ CINNAMON

Pantry Essentials

If you're serious about the anti-inflammatory diet, you will do well to make the following ingredients a staple in your pantry:

Canned Items

- Tomatoes, crushed
- Tomatoes, chopped
- Red bell peppers, roasted, in oil
- Coconut milk, lite
- Broth, vegetable, no salt added
- Broth, chicken, no salt added

Herbs And Spices

- Turmeric, ground
- Thyme, dried
- Salt, Himalayan pink or sea

- Rosemary, dried
- Red pepper flakes
- Peppercorns
- Oregano, dried
- Onion powder
- Nutmeg, ground
- Ginger, ground
- Garlic powder
- Curry powder
- Cinnamon, ground
- Chili powder

Nuts, Seeds, Legumes, And Grains

- Sunflower seeds
- Sesame seeds, toasted
- Rice, brown, cooked
- Quinoa
- Peanut butter
- Lentils, canned
- Chickpeas, canned
- Beans, kidney, canned
- Beans, black, canned
- Almond butter

Oils, Vinegars, And Condiments

- Vinegar, apple cider
- Soy sauce, low-sodium (or gluten-free or tamari)
- Olive oil, extra-virgin
- Mustard, Dijon

Sugar, Baking Ingredients, And Flours

- Vanilla extract
- Sugar, brown
- Stevia
- Milk, almond, hemp, or rice, unsweetened
- Maple syrup, pure

- Honey
- Green tea
- Cocoa powder, unsweetened
- Arrowroot powder (or cornstarch)

Tips And Tricks

Here are a few suggestions I give to my clients to make it easier for them to cook the food, and stick to the diet:

- Weekly Diet Plans Work. If you think too much ahead, things will be hard. Plan for a week, or even less. Make a meal plan using the recipes in this book, and make a shopping list. Shopping only for the ingredients you'll be using in the following week will ensure that they stay fresh, and your brain stays relatively stress-free.
- Cook in Large Batches. If you're lazy like me and wouldn't like to cook three times every day, try cooking a LOT. This only works for dishes that store well in the fridge. Take a serving size out of the fridge, heat using a microwave, eat, repeat.
- Have Fun With Leftovers. Leftovers are a great opportunity to let your imagination run wild and invent a new recipe tailored to your personal taste!
- Veggies are Love. Buy lots of fresh vegetables when you're at a grocery store. Better yet, take a stroll through a farmers' market near you.
- Try Different Cooking Methods. Depending on how much time you have, and when you want to eat, a different cooking method might make the work easier. Slow cooking, for example, is great for someone who has a day job and would like to come back home to a home cooked meal, without another home cook.
- Prepare and Shop on Weekends and Holidays. If you have a full time job, make sure you take care of some of the planning and shopping on the day off.
- Frozen veggies and fruits are Great. There is a misconception that frozen fruits and vegetables lose their nutrition. That is just not true. These are usually flash frozen while they are at their peak of ripeness, and due to being frozen, that peak is maintained for much longer!

- Machine Tools are Handy. Food processors are love, Food processors are life.
- Store Food Right. Different ingredients like to be stored in different ways. While an ingredient is best stored in the freezer, another might do stored at room temperature. If you're not sure about the best way to store a particular ingredient, google is your friend!
- Internet for The Win. If you can't find that pesky ingredient in a nearby store, check online on amazon. If you can't figure out a cooking procedure by words alone, watch a YouTube video.

About The Recipes

All right! I think we are done with the basics. Let us dive into the recipes! Make sure you read the ingredients and directions carefully before starting a recipe. This book calls for all kinds of tools ranging from slow cookers to instant pots. If you don't have the appliance required to cook a particular recipe, just skip to a different recipe, and return to it once you have invested in the appliance. Also, Make sure you're not allergic to any of the ingredients. Let's go!

Smoothies and Drinks
Almond Blueberry Smoothie
Time To Prepare: ten minutes
Time to Cook: 0 minutes
Yield: Servings 1
Ingredients:

- 1 banana
- 1 cup frozen blueberries
- 1 tbsp. almond butter
- 1/2 cup almond milk
- Water, as required

Directions:

1. Put in everything to a blender jug.
2. Cover the jug firmly.
3. Blend until the desired smoothness is achieved. Serve and enjoy!

Nutritional Info: Calories: 211 ‖ Fat: 0.2 g ‖ Protein: 5.6 g ‖ Carbohydrates: 3.4 g ‖ Fiber: 2.3 g

Almond Butter Smoothies
Time To Prepare: five minutes
Time to Cook: 0 minutes
Yield: Servings 1
Ingredients:

- 1 banana, if possible frozen for a creamier shake
- 1 cup of hemp milk
- 1 scoop of hemp protein
- 1 Tablespoon natural almond butter
- few ice cubes

Directions:
Blend all ingredients together and enjoy!

Nutritional Info: Calories: 533 kcal ‖ Protein: 31.23 g ‖ Fat: 26.31 g ‖ Carbohydrates: 47.13 g

Apple Cinnamon Water
Time To Prepare: five minutes
Time to Cook: five minutes
Yield: Servings 4
Ingredients:

- 1 whole apple, diced
- 5 cinnamon sticks
- Water to cover contents

Directions:

1. Put ingredients in the steamer basket. Put in pot.
2. Put in water cover contents.
3. Secure the lid. Cook on HIGH pressure five minutes.
4. When done, depressurize swiftly.
5. Remove steamer basket. Discard cooked produce.
6. Let flavored water cool. Chill completely before you serve.

Nutritional Info: Calories: 194 ‖ Fat: 0g ‖ Carbohydrates: 12g ‖ Protein: 0g

Baby Kale Pineapple Smoothie
Time To Prepare: five minutes
Time to Cook: 0 minutes
Yield: Servings 1
Ingredients:

- 1 cup almond milk
- 1 cup Kale
- 1 tablespoon hemp protein powder
- 1/2 cup frozen pineapple

Directions:
Put the almond milk, pineapple, and greens in the blender and blend until the desired smoothness is achieved.

Nutritional Info: Calories: 389 kcal ‖ Protein: 20.29 g ‖ Fat: 16.2 g ‖ Carbohydrates: 42.29 g

Beet and Cherry Smoothie
Time To Prepare: five minutes
Time to Cook: 0 minutes
Yield: Servings 4
Ingredients:

- ½ cup frozen cherries, pitted
- ½ teaspoon frozen banana
- 1 tablespoon almond butter
- 10-ounce almond milk, unsweetened
- 2 small beets, peeled and slice into four

Directions:

1. Put in all ingredients in a blender.
2. Blend until the desired smoothness is achieved.

Nutritional Info: Calories 470 ‖ Carbohydrates: 24 g ‖ Fat: 38 g ‖ Protein: 16 g

Beet Smoothie
Time To Prepare: ten minutes
Time to Cook: 0 minutes
Yield: Servings 2

Ingredients:

- 1 tbsp. almond butter
- 1/2 banana, peeled and frozen
- 1/2 cup cherries, pitted
- 10 oz. almond milk, unsweetened
- 2 beets, peeled and quartered

Directions:

1. In your blender, combine the milk with the beets, banana, cherries, and butter.
2. Pulse thoroughly, pour into glasses, before you serve. Enjoy!

Nutritional Info: Calories: 165 ‖ Fat: 5 g ‖ Protein: 5 g ‖ Carbohydrates: 22 g ‖ Fiber: 6 g

Berry Shrub
Time To Prepare: ten minutes
Time to Cook: twenty minutes
Yield: Servings 4
Ingredients:

- ½ a cup of chopped fresh oregano
- 1 cup of dried elderberries
- 2 cups of apple cider vinegar
- 2 cups of honey
- 2 cups of water

Directions:

1. Put in listed ingredients to the instant pot.
2. Secure the lid. Cook on HIGH pressure twenty minutes.
3. When done, depressurize naturally.
4. Pour ingredients through a sieve into a jar.
5. Let cool down. Chill.

Nutritional Info: Calories: 127 ‖ Fat: 0g ‖ Carbohydrates: 6g ‖ Protein: 0g

Blackberry & Ginger Milkshake

Time To Prepare: five minutes
Time to Cook: 0 minutes
Yield: Servings 2
Ingredients:

- 1 thumb-sized piece of ginger, grated
- 2 cups of almond milk
- 2 cups of blackberries, washed
- 2 cups of chopped peaches

Directions:

1. Combine all ingredients to a blender or juicer and blend until the desired smoothness is achieved.
2. Serve with a scattering of fresh blackberries and enjoy!

Nutritional Info: Calories: 619 kcal ‖ Protein: fifteen.42 g ‖ Fat: 11.63 g ‖ Carbohydrates: 123.04 g

Blackberry Italian Drink
Time To Prepare: five minutes
Time to Cook: fifteen minutes
Yield: Servings 4
Ingredients:

- 1 bottle sparkling water
- 1 cup blackberries
- 1 lemon, cut
- 2 tbsp. honey

Directions:

1. Put in 1 cup (non-carbonated) water to the instant pot.
2. Put in blackberries to the instant pot.
3. Secure the lid. Cook on HIGH pressure ten minutes.
4. When done, depressurize naturally.
5. Mash the berries in the instant pot. Move to dish. Let cool.
6. As blackberries cook, in a separate small deep cooking pan with a heavy bottom. Put in honey. Simmer five minutes. Cool down.

7. To make the drink. Ladle 1 teaspoon honey. Pour in fruit mixture. Put in carbonated water. Stir.

Nutritional Info: Calories: 249 ‖ Fat: 0.6g ‖ Carbohydrates: 55g ‖ Protein: 7.5g

Blended Coconut Milk and Banana Breakfast Smoothie
Time To Prepare: ten minutes
Time to Cook: 0 minutes
Yield: Servings 4
Ingredients:

- 2 cups almond milk
- 2 cups coconut milk
- 4 ripe moderate-sized bananas
- 4 tbsp. flax seeds
- 4 tsp. cinnamon

Directions:

1. Peel the banana and cut it into ½-inch pieces. Put all the ingredients in the blender and blend into a smoothie.
2. Put in a dash of cinnamon at the top of the smoothie before you serve.

Nutritional Info: Calories: 332 kcal ‖ Protein: 12.49 g ‖ Fat: 14.42 g ‖ Carbohydrates: 42.46 g

Blueberry And Spinach Shake
Time To Prepare: five minutes
Time to Cook: 0 minutes
Yield: Servings 2
Ingredients:

- 1 cup of low-fat Greek yogurt (not necessary)
- 1 cup of organic blueberries (or washed if non-organic)
- 1/2 cup of spinach
- ice cubes to the desired concentration

Directions:

1. Put in ingredients together in a blender until the desired smoothness is achieved and then serve in a tall glass.
2. Drizzle a few fresh berries on top if you prefer!

Nutritional Info: Calories: 233 kcal ‖ Protein: 10.68 g ‖ Fat: 5.38 g ‖ Carbohydrates: 37.13 g

Blueberry Lime Juice
Time To Prepare: five minutes
Time to Cook: five minutes
Yield: Servings 4
Ingredients:

- 1 cup fresh blueberries
- Water to cover contents
- Zest and juice of 1 lime

Directions:

1. Put ingredients in a mesh steamer basket for instant pot. Put in pot.
2. Pour in water to immerse contents.
3. Secure the lid. Cook on HIGH pressure five minutes.
4. When done, depressurize swiftly.
5. Remove steamer basket. Discard cooked produce.
6. Let flavored water cool. Chill completely before you serve.

Nutritional Info: Calories: 86 ‖ Fat: 0g ‖ Carbohydrates: 22g ‖ Protein: 0g

Blueberry Matcha Smoothie
Time To Prepare: five minutes
Time to Cook: 0 minutes
Yield: Servings 2
Ingredients:

- ¼ Teaspoon Ground Cinnamon
- ¼ Teaspoon Ground Ginger
- 1 Banana
- 1 Tablespoon Chia Seeds
- 1 Tablespoon Matcha Powder

- 2 Cups Almond Milk
- 2 Cups Blueberries, Frozen
- 2 Tablespoons Protein Powder, Optional
- A Pinch Sea Salt

Directions:
Blend all ingredients until the desired smoothness is achieved.

Nutritional Info: Calories: 208 ‖ Protein: 8.7 Grams ‖ Fat: 5.7 Grams ‖ Carbohydrates: 31 Grams

Blueberry Pomegranate Smoothie
Time To Prepare: five minutes
Time to Cook: 0 minutes
Yield: Servings 2
Ingredients:

- ¼ cup of canned coconut milk
- 1 cup of pomegranate juice, unsweetened
- 1 tbsp. of hemp seeds
- 2 cup of frozen blueberries
- 6 to 8 ice cubes

Directions:

1. Mix the smoothie ingredients in your high-speed blender.
2. Pulse the ingredients a few times to cut them up.
3. Combine the mixture on the highest speed setting for thirty to 60 seconds.
4. Pour into glasses and serve.

Nutritional Info: Calories: 282 kcal ‖ Protein: 5.64 g ‖ Fat: 13.8 g ‖ Carbohydrates: 37.75 g

Blueberry Smoothie
Time To Prepare: ten minutes
Time to Cook: 0 minutes
Yield: Servings 1
Ingredients:

- 1 banana, peeled
- 1 tbsp. almond butter

- 1 tsp. maca powder
- 1/2 cup almond milk, unsweetened
- 1/2 cup blueberries
- 1/2 cup water
- 1/4 tsp. ground cinnamon
- 2 handfuls baby spinach

Directions:

1. In your blender, combine the spinach with the banana, blueberries, almond butter, cinnamon, maca powder, water, and milk.
2. Pulse thoroughly, pour into a glass, before you serve. Enjoy!

Nutritional Info: Calories: 341 ‖ Fat: 12 g ‖ Protein: 10 g ‖ Carbohydrates: 54 g ‖ Fiber: 12 g

Broccoli Smoothie
Time To Prepare: *five minutes*
Time to Cook: *0 minutes*
Yield: Servings 4
Ingredients:

- 1 ½ cups strawberries
- 1 ½ cups water
- 1 cup broccoli florets
- 1 cup chopped spinach
- 2 bananas, cut, frozen
- 2 cups frozen mango chunks
- 2 cups pineapple juice

Directions:

1. Combine all ingredients into a blender and blend until the desired smoothness is achieved.
2. Pour into 4 tall glasses before you serve.

Nutritional Info: Calories: 222 kcal ‖ Protein: 3.51 g ‖ Fat: 1.98 g ‖ Carbohydrates: 51.45 g

Carrot and Orange Turmeric Drink

Time To Prepare: five minutes
Time to Cook: 0 minutes
Yield: Servings 2
Ingredients:

- 1 cup orange juice
- 1 tbsp. lemon juice
- 1/2 inch ginger slice
- 1/4 tsp. turmeric powder
- 2 carrots, peeled, chopped
- 2 tbsp. sugar

Directions:

1. In a blender, put in orange juice, sugar, turmeric powder, carrots, and lemon juice.
2. Blend well.

Serve!

Nutritional Info: Calories: 153 kcal ‖ Protein: 4.47 g ‖ Fat: 3.3 g ‖ Carbohydrates: 27.02 g

Cherry Smoothie
Time To Prepare: five minutes
Time to Cook: 0 minutes
Yield: Servings 4-6
Ingredients:

- 1 ½ cups vanilla Greek yogurt
- 2 bananas, cut
- 3 cups cherry juice
- 3 cups pitted, froze dark sweet cherries
- Fresh cherries, pitted
- Mint sprigs
- To decorate: Optional

Directions:

1. Combine all ingredients into a blender and blend until the desired smoothness is achieved.

2. Pour into 4 tall glasses.
3. Decorate using optional ingredients if using before you serve.

Nutritional Info: Calories: 114 kcal ‖ Protein: 2.36 g ‖ Fat: 1.88 g ‖ Carbohydrates: 23.49 g

Chocolate Cherry Smoothie
Time To Prepare: five minutes
Time to Cook: 0 minutes
Yield: Servings 2
Ingredients:

- 2 cups almond milk, unsweetened
- 2 dates, pitted, chopped or 2 teaspoons pure maple syrup
- 2 scoops protein powder or 4 tablespoons almond butter (not necessary)
- 4 cups pitted, frozen cherries
- 4 tablespoons cocoa or cacao powder
- Cacao nibs
- Granola
- Hemp hearts
- To serve: Optional

Directions:

1. Combine all ingredients into a blender and blend until the desired smoothness is achieved.
2. Pour into 2 tall glasses and serve topped with optional ingredients.

Nutritional Info: Calories: 339 kcal ‖ Protein: 16.37 g ‖ Fat: 21.34 g ‖ Carbohydrates: 27.99 g

Chocolate Latte with Reishi
Time To Prepare: five minutes
Time to Cook: ten minutes
Yield: Servings 2
Ingredients:

- 1 teaspoon Reishi powder
- 2 tablespoons coconut butter

- 4 cups almond milk, unsweetened
- 4 teaspoons raw cacao powder
- A pinch ground cinnamon
- A pinch sea salt
- Sweetener of your choice

Directions:

1. Put in almond milk into a deep cooking pan. Put the deep cooking pan using low heat.
2. When the milk is warm and just starts to bubble, remove the heat. Move into a blender.
3. Put in the remaining ingredients and blend for 30 – 40 seconds or until the desired smoothness is achieved.
4. Pour into mugs before you serve.

Nutritional Info: Calories: 461 kcal ‖ Protein: 19.32 g ‖ Fat: 30.57 g ‖ Carbohydrates: 28.08 g

Cooked Iced Tea
Time To Prepare: two minutes
Time to Cook: 4 minutes
Yield: Servings 4
Ingredients:

- 2 tbsp. honey
- 4 regular tea bags
- 6 cups water

Directions:

1. Put in ingredients to the instant pot.
2. Secure the lid. Cook on HIGH pressure 4 minutes.
3. When done, depressurize naturally.
4. Allow to cool to room temperature. Serve over ice.

Nutritional Info: Calories: 22 ‖ Fat: 0g ‖ Carbohydrates: 6g ‖ Protein: 0g

Cucumber Kiwi Green Smoothie
Time To Prepare: five minutes

Time to Cook: 0 minutes
Yield: Servings 2
Ingredients:

- ¼ cup of canned coconut milk
- 1 cup of coconut water
- 1 cup of seedless cucumber, chopped
- 2 ripe kiwi fruit
- 2 tbsps. of fresh chopped cilantro
- 6 to 8 ice cubes
- ice cubes

Directions:

1. Mix the smoothie ingredients in your high-speed blender.
2. Pulse the ingredients a few times to cut them up.
3. Combine the mixture on the highest speed setting for thirty to 60 seconds.
4. Pour into glasses and serve.

Nutritional Info: Calories: 140 kcal ‖ Protein: 5.1 g ‖ Fat: 10.52 g ‖ Carbohydrates: 7.4 g

Cucumber Melon Smoothie
Time To Prepare: five minutes
Time to Cook: 0 minutes
Yield: Servings 2
Ingredients:

- 1 ½ cups of chopped honeydew
- 1 cup of chilled coconut water
- 1 cup of seedless cucumber, diced
- 2 tbsp. of fresh mint
- 6 to 8 ice cubes

Directions:

1. Mix the smoothie ingredients in your high-speed blender.
2. Pulse the ingredients a few times to cut them up.
3. Combine the mixture on the highest speed setting for thirty to

60 seconds.
4. Pour into glasses and serve.

Nutritional Info: Calories: 300 kcal ‖ Protein: 5.83 g ‖ Fat: 8.55 g ‖ Carbohydrates: 51.21 g

Dreamy Yummy Orange Cream Smoothie
Time To Prepare: five minutes
Time to Cook: 0 minutes
Yield: Servings 2
Ingredients:

- ¼ cup of fresh orange juice
- ½ cup of canned full-fat coconut milk
- 1 cup of almond milk
- 1 navel orange, peel removed
- 6 to 8 ice cubes

Directions:

1. Mix the smoothie ingredients in your high-speed blender.
2. Pulse the ingredients a few times to cut them up.
3. Combine the mixture on the highest speed setting for thirty to 60 seconds.
4. Pour into glasses and serve.

Nutritional Info: Calories: 269 kcal ‖ Protein: 8.63 g ‖ Fat: 21.36 g ‖ Carbohydrates: 12.75 g

Fig Smoothie
Time To Prepare: five minutes
Time to Cook: 0 minutes
Yield: Servings 2
Ingredients:

- 1 Banana
- 1 Cup Almond Milk
- 1 Cup Whole Milk Yogurt, Plain
- 1 Tablespoon Almond Butter
- 1 Teaspoon Flaxseed, Ground
- 1 Teaspoon Honey, Raw

- 3-4 Ice Cubes
- 7 Figs, Halved (Fresh or Frozen)

Directions:

Blend all together ingredients until the desired smoothness is achieved, and serve instantly.

Nutritional Info: Calories: 362 ‖ Protein: 9 Grams ‖ Fat: 12 Grams ‖ Carbohydrates: 60 Grams

Flu Fighting Tonic
Time To Prepare: five minutes
Time to Cook: ten minutes
Yield: Servings 2
Ingredients:

- ½ teaspoon turmeric powder
- 2 tablespoons clear honey if possible manuka
- Boiling water, as required
- Juice of 2 lemons
- Lemon slices to decorate

Directions:

1. Split the lemon juice into 2 mugs. Put in ¼ teaspoon turmeric powder into each mug.
2. Put in a tablespoon of honey into each mug.
3. Pour boiling water to fill up the mugs. Stir.
4. Decorate using a slice of lemon before you serve.

Nutritional Info: Calories: 123 kcal ‖ Protein: 3.59 g ‖ Fat: 3.23 g ‖ Carbohydrates: 22.78 g

Fresh Cranberry And Lime Juice
Time To Prepare: five minutes
Time to Cook: 0 minutes
Yield: Servings 2
Ingredients:

- 1/2½ cups of mixed berries (frozen are fine)
- 1/2½ cups of spinach
- 2 limes, juiced

- 4 cups of cranberries

Directions:
Mix all the ingredients with water in a juicer until pureed and serve instantly over ice.

Nutritional Info: Calories: 578 kcal ‖ Protein: 6.83 g ‖ Fat: 9.92 g ‖ Carbohydrates: 119.35 g

Fresh Tropical Juice
Time To Prepare: five minutes
Time to Cook: 0 minutes
Yield: Servings 2
Ingredients:

- 1 whole pineapple, peeled and slice into chunks.
- 1 cup of water
- 1/2 can of low-fat coconut milk

Directions:

1. Put in all ingredients to a juicer and blend until the desired smoothness is achieved.
2. Serve over ice.

Nutritional Info: Calories: 116 kcal ‖ Protein: 3.72 g ‖ Fat: 3.13 g ‖ Carbohydrates: 19.55 g

Ginger Ale
Time To Prepare: five minutes
Time to Cook: thirty minutes
Yield: Servings 4
Ingredients:

- 1 pound fresh ginger, unpeeled, diced
- 1 quart carbonated water
- 1 tbsp. honey
- Ice for serving
- Juice and rind of 2 lemons
- Lime wedges

Directions:

1. Put ginger and lemon juice in a food processor. Pulse to smooth consistency.
2. Move puree to the instant pot. Mix in honey.
3. Put in lemon peel to the instant pot.
4. Secure the lid. Cook on HIGH pressure thirty minutes.
5. When done, depressurize naturally. Strain and chill.
6. Serve over ice.

Nutritional Info: Calories: 108 ‖ Fat: 0g ‖ Carbohydrates: 28g ‖ Protein: 0g

Ginger, Carrot, and Turmeric Smoothie
Time To Prepare: five minutes
Time to Cook: 0 minutes
Yield: Servings 2
Ingredients:

- ½ cup Mango, fresh or frozen chunks
- 1 big Carrot, peeled and chopped
- 1 cup Coconut water
- 1 Orange, peeled and separated
- 1 tbsp. Hemp seeds, raw, shelled
- 1 tsp. Ginger, ground
- 1 tsp. Turmeric, ground
- 1/8 tsp. Cayenne pepper

Directions:
Puree all of the ingredients with one-half cup of ice until the desired smoothness is achieved and drink instantly.

Nutritional Info: Calories 250 ‖ 35 grams sugar ‖ 4.5 grams fat ‖ 7 grams fiber ‖ 48 grams carbs ‖ 6 grams protein

Golden Chai Latte
Time To Prepare: five minutes
Time to Cook: ten minutes
Yield: Servings 2
Ingredients:

- ¼ teaspoon ground cinnamon
- ½ cup water
- ½ tablespoon maple syrup

- ½ tablespoon turmeric powder
- 1 ¼ cups cashew milk or any other non-dairy milk of your choice
- 1 teaspoon loose leaf chai tea
- 1/8 teaspoon ground nutmeg
- A pinch ground cardamom

Directions:

1. Put in water and 1-cup milk into a deep cooking pan. Put the deep cooking pan on moderate heat.
2. Put in chai leaves in a tea strainer (the type that that has a lid and you can close). Lower the strainer in the deep cooking pan. Put in spices.
3. When it just comes to a light boil, remove the heat. Allow it to cool for five minutes. Take out the tea strainer and discard the leaves.
4. Put in maple syrup and stir.
5. Pour into glasses. Sprinkle remaining cashew milk on top. Decorate using cinnamon and nutmeg before you serve.

Nutritional Info: Calories: 142 kcal ‖ Protein: 8.59 g ‖ Fat: 6.26 g ‖ Carbohydrates: 13.3 g

Green Vanilla Smoothie
Time To Prepare: ten minutes
Time to Cook: o minutes
Yield: Servings 1
Ingredients:

- 1 1/2 cups fresh spinach leaves
- 1 banana, cut in chunks
- 1 cup grapes
- 1 tub (6 oz.) vanilla yogurt
- 1/2 apple, cored and chopped

Directions:

1. Put in everything to a blender jug.
2. Cover the jug firmly.

3. Blend until the desired smoothness is achieved. Serve and enjoy!

Nutritional Info: Calories: 131 ‖ Fat: 0.2 g ‖ Protein: 2.6 g ‖ Carbohydrates: 9.1 g ‖ Fiber: 1.3 g

Hibiscus Tea
Time To Prepare: five minutes
Time to Cook: ten minutes
Yield: Servings 4
Ingredients:

- 1 tbsp. honey
- 1 tsp fresh ginger, grated
- 10 cups water
- 2 cup dried hibiscus petals
- Rind from 1 pineapple

Directions:

1. Wash hibiscus leaves meticulously with cold water.
2. Take away the dust.
3. Put in water, honey, and ginger to the instant pot. Stir.
4. Mix in hibiscus petals and pineapple rind.
5. Secure the lid. Cook on HIGH pressure ten minutes.
6. When done, depressurize naturally.
7. Remove pineapple rind. Pass liquid through a fine-mesh strainer.
8. Cool thoroughly. Chill before you serve.

Nutritional Info: Calories: 114 ‖ Fat: 0g ‖ Carbohydrates: 28g ‖ Protein: 0g

Hot Apple Cider
Time To Prepare: five minutes
Time to Cook: fifteen minutes
Yield: Servings 4
Ingredients:

- ½ cup fresh cranberries
- ½ cup honey

- ½ star of anise
- ½ tsp whole cloves
- 1 lemon, peeled, cut into segments
- 1 orange, peeled, cut into segments
- 2 cinnamon sticks
- 7 medium apples, cored, quarter
- Water to cover ingredients

Directions:

1. Put in apples, lemon, orange, and cranberries to the instant pot.
2. Put in cinnamon stick, star anise, and cloves.
3. Pour in water to immerse ingredients.
4. Secure the lid. Cook on HIGH pressure fifteen minutes.
5. Depressurize naturally.
6. Mash fruit using a masher to release juices.
7. Strain the liquid. Chill completely before you serve.

Nutritional Info: Calories: 153 ‖ Fat: 9g ‖ Carbohydrates: 14g ‖ Protein: 4g

Hot Peppermint Vanilla Latte
Time To Prepare: *five minutes*
Time to Cook: *five minutes*
Yield: Servings 4
Ingredients:

- ¼ cup honey
- 1 tsp vanilla
- 2 cups coffee
- 23 drops peppermint oil
- 4 cups almond milk

Directions:

1. Put in listed ingredients to the instant pot.
2. Secure the lid. Cook on HIGH pressure five minutes.
3. When done, depressurize naturally.
4. Serve warm.

Nutritional Info: Calories: 279 ‖ Fat: 3g ‖ Carbohydrates: 61g ‖ Protein: 3g

Instant Horchata
Time To Prepare: *five minutes*
Time to Cook: *five minutes*
Yield: Servings 4
Ingredients:

- 1 cinnamon stick, broken into little chunks
- 32 ounces rice milk
- 6 tbsp. honey

Directions:

1. Put in listed ingredients to the instant pot.
2. Secure the lid. Cook on HIGH pressure five minutes.
3. When done, depressurize naturally over ten minutes.
4. Cool thoroughly. Chill before you serve.

Nutritional Info: Calories: 226 ‖ Fat: 1g ‖ Carbohydrates: 53g ‖ Protein: 2g

Jamaican Hibiscus Tea
Time To Prepare: *five minutes*
Time to Cook: *five minutes*
Yield: Servings 4
Ingredients:

- ½ tsp ginger, minced
- 1 cup dried hibiscus flowers
- 1 tbsp. honey
- 8 cups water
- Ice as required
- Juice of 1 lime

Directions:

1. Put in hibiscus flowers, water, honey, and ginger to the instant pot.
2. Secure the lid. Cook on HIGH pressure five minutes.

3. When done, depressurize naturally.
4. Cool thoroughly. Move to glass decanter. Mix in lime Juice. Pour over ice.

Nutritional Info: Calories: 197 ‖ Fat: 0g ‖ Carbohydrates: 18g ‖ Protein: 0g

Kale Smoothie
Time To Prepare: ten minutes
Time to Cook: 0 minutes
Yield: Servings 2
Ingredients:

- 10 kale leaves
- 2 pears, chopped
- 5 bananas, peeled and slice into chunks
- 5 cups almond milk
- 5 tbsp. almond butter

Directions:

1. In your blender, combine the kale with the bananas, pears, almond butter, and almond milk.
2. Pulse thoroughly, split into glasses, before you serve. Enjoy!

Nutritional Info: Calories: 267 ‖ Fat: 11 g ‖ Protein: 7 g ‖ Carbohydrates: fifteen g ‖ Fiber: 7 g

Kiwi Strawberry Smoothie
Time To Prepare: ten minutes
Time to Cook: 0 minutes
Yield: Servings 1
Ingredients:

- ¼ cup Chia seed powder
- ½ cup Strawberries, fresh or frozen, chopped
- 1 Banana, diced
- 1 cup Milk, almond or coconut
- 1 Kiwi, peeled and chopped
- 1 tsp. Basil, ground
- 1 tsp. Turmeric, ground

Directions:
Drink instantly after all the ingredients have been thoroughly combined.

Nutritional Info: Calories 250 ‖ 9.9 grams sugar ‖ 1 gram fat ‖ 34 grams carbs ‖ 4.3 grams fiber ‖

Lemon Ginger Iced Tea
Time To Prepare: five minutes
Time to Cook: ten minutes
Yield: Servings 2-3
Ingredients:

- ¼ teaspoon turmeric
- 1 tablespoon fresh lemon juice or to taste (not necessary)
- 1 tablespoon maple syrup
- 2 – 3 lemon slices
- 2 inches fresh ginger, peeled, thinly cut or to taste
- 3-4 cups water
- A pinch ground cinnamon

Directions:

1. Pour water into a deep cooking pan. Put in ginger, turmeric, lemon slices, and cinnamon. Put the deep cooking pan on moderate heat.
2. Cover and simmer for eight - ten minutes.
3. Strain and pour into a jar. Place the maple syrup, and lemon juice, then stir. Chill for eight – 10 hours.
4. Stir thoroughly. Pour into glasses before you serve.

Nutritional Info: Calories: 55 kcal ‖ Protein: 2.32 g ‖ Fat: 2.13 g ‖ Carbohydrates: 7.47 g

Mango and Ginger Infused Water
Time To Prepare: five minutes
Time to Cook: five minutes
Yield: Servings 4
Ingredients:

- 1 cup fresh mango, chopped
- 2-inch piece ginger, peeled, cubed

- Water to cover ingredients

Directions:

1. Put ingredients in the mesh steamer basket.
2. Put basket in the instant pot.
3. Put in water to immerse contents.
4. Secure the lid. Cook on HIGH pressure five minutes.
5. When done, depressurize swiftly.
6. Remove steamer basket. Discard cooked produce.
7. Let flavored water cool. Chill completely and serve.

Nutritional Info: Calories: 209 ‖ Fat: 1g ‖ Carbohydrates: 51g ‖ Protein: 2g

Mango Tomato Smoothie
Time To Prepare: five minutes
Time to Cook: 0 minutes
Yield: Servings 4
Ingredients:

- 1 cup almond milk
- 2 cups chopped cilantro
- 2 cups pineapple chunks
- 2 mangoes, peeled, pitted
- 4 Campari tomatoes, chopped
- 6 cups fresh baby spinach

Directions:

1. Combine all ingredients into a blender and blend until the desired smoothness is achieved.
2. Pour into 4 tall glasses before you serve.

Nutritional Info: Calories: 395 kcal ‖ Protein: 13.1 g ‖ Fat: 8.19 g ‖ Carbohydrates: 73.65 g

Mixed Fruit & Nut Milkshake
Time To Prepare: five minutes
Time to Cook: 0 minutes
Yield: Servings 2

Ingredients:

- I tbsp. of honey
- 1/2 cup of almond milk
- 1½ grapefruit; peeled and chopped
- 1/2½ inch piece of ginger, minced
- 12 strawberries
- 2 tbsp. of chopped almonds
- juice of I orange

Directions:

1. Put everything but the strawberries in a blender until the desired smoothness is achieved.
2. Put in in the strawberries and blend until pureed, serving in a tall glass.

Nutritional Info: Calories: 140 kcal ‖ Protein: 5.89 g ‖ Fat: 5.84 g ‖ Carbohydrates: 17.36 g

Parsley Ginger Green Juice
Time To Prepare: five minutes
Time to Cook: o minutes
Yield: Servings 2
Ingredients:

- 2 cucumbers, chopped
- 2 green apples, cored
- 2 lemons, peeled, halved
- 4 cups chopped parsley
- 4 cups chopped spinach
- 4 inches fresh ginger, peeled, cut
- 6 stalks celery, chopped

Directions:

1. Juice together all the ingredients in a juicer.
2. Pour into 2 glasses before you serve.

Nutritional Info: Calories: 239 kcal ‖ Protein: 10.74 g ‖ Fat: 5.08 g ‖

Carbohydrates: 44.86 g

Peach And Raspberry Lemonade
Time To Prepare: *five minutes*
Time to Cook: *five minutes*
Yield: Servings 4
Ingredients:

- ½ cup fresh raspberries
- 1 cup fresh peaches, chopped
- Water to cover ingredients
- Zest and juice of 1 lemon

Directions:

1. Put ingredients in mesh basket for instant pot. Put in pot.
2. Put in water to barely cover the fruit.
3. Secure the lid. Cook on HIGH pressure five minutes.
4. When done, depressurize swiftly.
5. Remove steamer basket. Discard cooked produce.
6. Let flavored water cool. Chill completely before you serve.

Nutritional Info: Calories: 77 ‖ Fat: 0g ‖ Carbohydrates: 19g ‖ Protein: 0g

Peach Maple Smoothie
Time To Prepare: *ten minutes*
Time to Cook: *o minutes*
Yield: Servings 1
Ingredients:

- 1 cup fat-free yogurt
- 1 cup ice
- 2 tbsp. maple syrup
- 4 big peaches, peeled and chopped

Directions:

1. Put in everything to a blender jug.
2. Cover the jug firmly.
3. Blend until the desired smoothness is achieved. Serve and

enjoy!

Nutritional Info: Calories: 125 ‖ Fat: 0.4 g ‖ Protein: 5.6 g ‖ Carbohydrates: 8 g ‖ Fiber: 2.3 g

Peachy Keen Smoothie
Time To Prepare: five minutes
Time to Cook: o minutes
Yield: Servings 2
Ingredients:

- 1 ½ cups of frozen peaches
- 1 cup of almond milk
- 1 small frozen banana
- 2 tbsp. of raw hemp seeds
- 6 to 8 ice cubes
- Pinch of ground ginger

Directions:

1. Mix the smoothie ingredients in your high-speed blender.
2. Pulse the ingredients a few times to cut them up.
3. Combine the mixture on the highest speed setting for thirty to 60 seconds.
4. Pour into glasses and serve.

Nutritional Info: Calories: 388 kcal ‖ Protein: 10.59 g ‖ Fat: 11.93 g ‖ Carbohydrates: 64.08 g

Pineapple & Ginger Juice
Time To Prepare: five minutes
Time to Cook: o minutes
Yield: Servings 2
Ingredients:

- 2 apples, cored, chopped
- 2 cucumbers, chopped
- 2 cups chopped pineapple
- 2 cups spinach
- 2 inches ginger, peeled, cut
- 2 lemons, peeled, halved

- 8 celery stalks, chopped

Directions:

1. Juice together all the ingredients in a juicer.
2. Pour into 2 glasses before you serve.

Nutritional Info: Calories: 339 kcal ‖ Protein: 7.44 g ‖ Fat: 4.23 g ‖ Carbohydrates: 75.38 g

Pineapple and Greens Smoothie
Time To Prepare: five minutes
Time to Cook: 0 minutes
Yield: Servings 2
Ingredients:

- ¾ cup of almond milk
- 1 cup of chopped spinach
- 1 cup of frozen pineapple
- 1 small frozen banana
- 1 tbsp. of honey
- 2 tbsp. Of chia seeds

Directions:

1. Mix the smoothie ingredients in your high-speed blender.
2. Pulse the ingredients a few times to cut them up.
3. Combine the mixture on the highest speed setting for thirty to 60 seconds.
4. Pour into glasses and serve.

Nutritional Info: Calories: 272 kcal ‖ Protein: 5.27 g ‖ Fat: 4.5 g ‖ Carbohydrates: 56.37 g

Pineapple- Ginger Smoothie
Time To Prepare: five minutes
Time to Cook: 0 minutes
Yield: Servings 1
Ingredients:

- ½ inch thick ginger, cut

- 1 cup coconut milk
- 1 cup pineapple slice

Directions:

1. Put all ingredients in a blender.
2. Pulse until the desired smoothness is achieved.
3. Chill before you serve.

Nutritional Info: Calories 299 ‖ Fat: 8 g ‖ Protein: 9 g ‖ Carbohydrates: 51 g

Pineapple Smoothie
Time To Prepare: ten minutes
Time to Cook: 0 minutes
Yield: Servings 2
Ingredients:

- 1 1/2 cups pineapple chunks
- 1 cup coconut water
- 1 orange, peeled and slice into quarters
- 1 tbsp. fresh grated ginger
- 1 tsp. chia seeds
- 1 tsp. turmeric powder
- A pinch black pepper

Directions:

1. In your blender, combine the coconut water with the orange, pineapple, ginger, chia seeds, turmeric, and black pepper.
2. Pulse thoroughly, pour into a glass.

Makes for a great breakfast!

Nutritional Info: Calories: 151 ‖ Fat: 2 g ‖ Protein: 4 g ‖ Carbohydrates: 12 g ‖ Fiber: 6 g

Pink California Smoothie
Time To Prepare: ten minutes
Time to Cook: 0 minutes
Yield: Servings 1
Ingredients:

- 1 container (8 oz.) lemon yogurt
- 1/3 cup orange juice
- 7 big strawberries

Directions:

1. Put in everything to a blender jug.
2. Cover the jug firmly.
3. Blend until the desired smoothness is achieved. Serve and enjoy!

Nutritional Info: Calories: 144 ‖ Fat: 0.4 g ‖ Protein: 5.6 g ‖ Carbohydrates: 8 g ‖ Fiber: 2.3 g

Pumpkin Pie Smoothie
Time To Prepare: five minutes
Time to Cook: 0 minutes
Yield: Servings 2
Ingredients:

- ½ Cup Pumpkin, Canned & Unsweetened
- 1 Banana
- 1 Cup Almond Milk
- 1 Teaspoon Ground Cinnamon
- 1 Teaspoon Ground Nutmeg
- 1 Teaspoon Maple Syrup, Pure
- 1 Teaspoon Vanilla Extract Pure
- 2 Tablespoons Almond Butter, Heaping
- 2-3 Ice Cubes

Directions:
Blend all ingredients together until the desired smoothness is achieved.

Nutritional Info: Calories: 235 ‖ Protein: 5.6 Grams ‖ Fat: 11 Grams ‖ Carbohydrates: 27.8 Grams

Purple Fruit Smoothie
Time To Prepare: ten minutes
Time to Cook: 0 minutes
Yield: Servings 1
Ingredients:

- 2 frozen bananas, cut in chunks
- 1 cup orange juice
- 1 tbsp. honey, optional
- 1 tsp. vanilla extract, optional
- 1/2 cup frozen blueberries

Directions:

1. Put in everything to a blender jug.
2. Cover the jug firmly.
3. Blend until the desired smoothness is achieved. Serve and enjoy!

Nutritional Info: Calories: 133 ‖ Fat: 1.1 g ‖ Protein: 3.6 g ‖ Carbohydrates: 7.6 g ‖ Fiber: 1.3 g

Raspberry Banana Smoothie
Time To Prepare: ten minutes
Time to Cook: 0 minutes
Yield: Servings 1
Ingredients:

- 1 banana
- 1 cup almond milk
- 1 cup frozen raspberries
- 1 cup raspberry yogurt
- 1 tbsp. flaxseed meal
- 1/4 cup Concord grape juice
- 1/4 cup rolled oats
- 16 whole almonds

Directions:

1. Put in everything to a blender jug.
2. Cover the jug firmly.
3. Blend until the desired smoothness is achieved and then serve. Enjoy!

Nutritional Info: Calories: 214 ‖ Fat: 0.4 g ‖ Protein: 5.6 g ‖ Carbohydrates: 8 g ‖ Fiber: 2.3 g

Raspberry Smoothie
Time To Prepare: ten minutes
Time to Cook: o minutes
Yield: Servings 2
Ingredients:

- 1 avocado, pitted and peeled
- 1/2 cup raspberries
- 3/4 cup raspberry juice
- 3/4 cup orange juice

Directions:

1. In your blender, combine the avocado with the raspberry juice, orange juice, and raspberries.
2. Pulse thoroughly, split into 2 glasses, before you serve. Enjoy!

Nutritional Info: Calories: 125 ‖ Fat: 11 g ‖ Protein: 3 g ‖ Carbohydrates: 9 g ‖ Fiber: 7 g

Spicy Tomato Smoothie
Time To Prepare: five minutes
Time to Cook: o minutes
Yield: Servings 2
Ingredients:

- ¼ cup chopped red onion
- 1 jalapeño, cut, deseed if you wish
- 1 small bunch cilantro, chopped
- 1 small cucumber
- 2 big carrots, chopped
- 2 cloves garlic, peeled
- 6 small vine tomatoes
- Juice of 2 limes

Directions:

1. Combine all ingredients into a blender and blend until the desired smoothness is achieved.
2. Pour into 2 tall glasses before you serve.

Nutritional Info: Calories: 269 kcal ‖ Protein: 24.87 g ‖ Fat: 8.71 g ‖ Carbohydrates: 26.89 g

Strawberry Oatmeal Smoothie
Time To Prepare: ten minutes
Time to Cook: 0 minutes
Yield: Servings 1
Ingredients:

- 1 cup soy milk
- 1 banana, broken into chunks
- 14 frozen strawberries
- 1/2 cup rolled oats
- 1/2 tsp. vanilla extract
- 1 1/2 tsp. honey

Directions:

1. Put in everything to a blender jug.
2. Cover the jug firmly.
3. Blend until the desired smoothness is achieved. Serve and enjoy!

Nutritional Info: Calories: 172 ‖ Fat: 0.4 g ‖ Protein: 5.6 g ‖ Carbohydrates: 8 g ‖ Fiber: 2 g

Sweet & Savoury Smoothie
Time To Prepare: five minutes
Time to Cook: 0 minutes
Yield: Servings 2
Ingredients:

- 1 apple, peeled and cut
- 1 banana, peeled and cut
- 1 cup of almond or soy milk
- 1 cup of fresh pineapple, peeled and cut
- 1 tbsp. of lemon juice
- 1/2 tbsp. of ginger, grated
- 1/4 tsp of ground turmeric
- 2 cups of carrots, peeled and cut
- 2 cups of filtered water.

Directions:

1. Blend carrots and water to make a pureed carrot juice.
2. Pour into a Mason jar or sealable container, cover, and store in the refrigerator.
3. When done, put in the rest of the smoothie ingredients to a blender or juicer until the desired smoothness is achieved.
4. Put in the carrot juice in at the end, blending meticulously until the desired smoothness is achieved.
5. Serve with or without ice.

Nutritional Info: Calories: 225 kcal ‖ Protein: 6.03 g ‖ Fat: 5.78 g ‖ Carbohydrates: 39.93 g

Sweet Cranberry Juice
Time To Prepare: five minutes
Time to Cook: 8 minutes
Yield: Servings 4
Ingredients:

- ½ cup honey
- 1 cinnamon stick
- 1 gallon filtered water
- 4 cups fresh cranberries
- Juice of 1 lemon

Directions:

1. Put in cranberries, ½ of water, cinnamon cling to the instant pot.
2. Secure the lid. Cook on HIGH pressure 8 minutes.
3. Depressurize naturally.
4. Once cool, strain liquid. Put in remaining water.
5. Mix in honey and lemon. Cool thoroughly.
6. Chill before you serve.

Nutritional Info: Calories: 184 ‖ Fat: 0g ‖ Carbohydrates: 49g ‖ Protein: 1g

Triple Fruit Smoothie
Time To Prepare: ten minutes

Time to Cook: o minutes
Yield: Servings 1
Ingredients:

- 1 banana, peeled and chopped
- 1 container (8 oz.) peach yogurt
- 1 cup ice cubes
- 1 cup strawberries
- 1 kiwi, cut
- 1/2 cup blueberries
- 1/2 cup orange juice

Directions:

1. Put in everything to a blender jug.
2. Cover the jug firmly.
3. Blend until the desired smoothness is achieved. Serve and enjoy!

Nutritional Info: Calories: 124 ‖ Fat: 0.4 g ‖ Protein: 5.6 g ‖ Carbohydrates: 8 g ‖ Fiber: 2.3 g

Tropical Mango Coconut Smoothie
Time To Prepare: five minutes
Time to Cook: o minutes
Yield: Servings 2
Ingredients:

- ½ cup of canned coconut milk
- ½ cup of fresh orange juice
- 1 ½ cups of frozen mango
- 1 ½ tsp of honey
- 1 medium frozen banana
- 1 tbsp. of fresh lemon juice

Directions:

1. Mix the smoothie ingredients in your high-speed blender.
2. Pulse the ingredients a few times to cut them up.

3. Combine the mixture on the highest speed setting for thirty to 60 seconds.
4. Pour into glasses and serve.

Nutritional Info: Calories: 354 kcal ‖ Protein: 6.7 g ‖ Fat: 18.09 g ‖ Carbohydrates: 47.42 g

Tropical Pineapple Kiwi Smoothie
Time To Prepare: five minutes
Time to Cook: 0 minutes
Yield: Servings 2
Ingredients:

- 1 ½ cup of frozen pineapple
- 1 cup of canned full-fat coconut milk
- 1 ripe kiwi; peeled and chopped
- 1 tsp of spirulina powder
- 3 tsp of lime juice
- 6 to 8 ice cubes

Directions:

1. Mix the smoothie ingredients in your high-speed blender.
2. Pulse the ingredients a few times to cut them up.
3. Combine the mixture on the highest speed setting.
4. Pour into glasses and serve.

Nutritional Info: Calories: 480 kcal ‖ Protein: 7.38 g ‖ Fat: 31.92 g ‖ Carbohydrates: 48.35 g

Turmeric and Ginger Tonic
Time To Prepare: five minutes
Time to Cook: ten minutes
Yield: Servings 4
Ingredients:

- 1/8 teaspoon cayenne pepper
- 2 tablespoons grated, fresh ginger
- 2 tablespoons grated, fresh turmeric
- 6 cups water
- Juice of 2 lemons

- Maple syrup or honey to taste
- The rind of 2 lemons, peeled

Directions:

1. Put in water, ginger, turmeric, cayenne pepper, and lemon rind into a deep cooking pan.
2. Put the deep cooking pan on moderate to high heat. (Do not boil)
3. Once the mixture is hot, remove from heat.
4. Strain into 4 mugs. Put in honey and lemon juice and stir.
5. Serve warm.

Nutritional Info: Calories: 48 kcal ‖ Protein: 2.28 g ‖ Fat: 1.81 g ‖ Carbohydrates: 7.03 g

Turmeric Delight
Time To Prepare: five minutes
Time to Cook: 0 minutes
Yield: Servings 2
Ingredients:

- ¼ Teaspoon Ginger
- ½ Teaspoon Cinnamon
- 1 Banana, Sliced
- 1 Tablespoon Lemon Juice, Fresh
- 1 Teaspoon Turmeric
- 2 Cups Yogurt, Plain & Whole Milk
- 2 Teaspoons Honey, Raw

Directions:

Combine all ingredients into a blender then blend until the desired smoothness is achieved.

Nutritional Info: Calories: 234 ‖ Protein: 9.3 Grams ‖ Fat: 8.2 Grams ‖ Carbohydrates: 33.5 Grams

Turmeric Hot Chocolate
Time To Prepare: five minutes
Time to Cook: ten minutes
Yield: Servings 2
Ingredients:

- 1/8 tsp. cayenne pepper, optional
- 1/8 tsp. pepper
- 2 cups milk
- 2 tsp. ground turmeric
- 3 tbsp. cacao or cocoa powder
- 4 tsp. coconut oil
- 4 tsp. honey

Directions:

1. Put in milk, turmeric, cocoa, and coconut oil into a deep cooking pan. Put the deep cooking pan on moderate heat. Coconut oil and pepper are added because it helps to absorb the turmeric.
2. Whisk regularly until well blended.
3. When it starts to boil, remove from heat. Put in honey, cayenne pepper, and pepper and whisk well.
4. Split into 2 cups before you serve.

Nutritional Info: Calories: 339 kcal ‖ Protein: 12.76 g ‖ Fat: 21.19 g ‖ Carbohydrates: 30.35 g

Turmeric Tea
Time To Prepare: five minutes
Time to Cook: fifteen minutes
Yield: Servings 2
Ingredients:

- ½ teaspoon ground ginger
- ½ teaspoon turmeric powder
- ½ tsp ground cinnamon
- 2 cups water
- 2 lemon juices
- 2 tablespoons honey

Directions:

1. Put in water into a deep cooking pan. Put the deep cooking pan on moderate heat.

2. When it starts to boil, put in turmeric, cinnamon, and ginger and stir slowly.
3. Remove the heat. Cover and allow the mixture to steep for 12 – fifteen minutes. Put in honey and lemon juice.
4. Stir and pour into mugs.
5. Serve.

Nutritional Info: Calories: 121 kcal ‖ Protein: 3.57 g ‖ Fat: 3.2 g ‖ Carbohydrates: 21.97 g

Vanilla Avocado Smoothie
Time To Prepare: ten minutes
Time to Cook: 0 minutes
Yield: Servings 1
Ingredients:

- 1 cup almond milk
- 1 ripe avocado, halved and pitted
- 1/2 cup vanilla yogurt
- 3 tbsp. honey
- 8 ice cubes

Directions:

1. Put in everything to a blender jug.
2. Cover the jug firmly.
3. Blend until the desired smoothness is achieved. Serve and enjoy!

Nutritional Info: Calories: 143 ‖ Fat: 1.2 g ‖ Protein: 4.6 g ‖ Carbohydrates: 21 g ‖ Fiber: 2.3 g

Vanilla Blueberry Smoothie
Time To Prepare: five minutes
Time to Cook: 0 minutes
Yield: Servings 1
Ingredients:

- 1 cup fresh blueberries
- 1 tbsp. flaxseed oil
- 2 cups hemp milk

- 2 tbsp. hemp protein powder
- Handful of ice/ 1 cup frozen blueberries

Directions:

1. Mix milk and fresh blueberries plus ice (or frozen blueberries) in a blender.
2. Blend for a minute, move to a glass, and mix in flaxseed oil.

Nutritional Info: Calories: 1041 kcal ‖ Protein: 35.21 g ‖ Fat: 41.04 g ‖ Carbohydrates: 140.4 g

Vanilla Turmeric Orange Juice
Time To Prepare: five minutes
Time to Cook: 0 minutes
Yield: Servings 2
Ingredients:

- ½ teaspoon turmeric powder
- 1 teaspoon ground cinnamon
- 2 cups unsweetened almond milk
- 2 teaspoons vanilla extract
- 6 oranges, peeled, separated into segments, deseeded
- Pepper to taste

Directions:

1. Juice the oranges. Put in the remaining ingredients.
2. Pour into 2 glasses before you serve.

Nutritional Info: Calories: 223 kcal ‖ Protein: 11.47 g ‖ Fat: 11.79 g ‖ Carbohydrates: fifteen.9 g

Voluptuous Vanilla Hot Drink
Time To Prepare: ten minutes
Time to Cook: 0 minutes
Yield: Servings 1
Ingredients:

- 1 scoop of hemp protein
- 1/2 Tbsp. ground cinnamon (or more to taste)

- 1/2 Tbsp. vanilla extract
- 3 cups unsweetened almond milk (or 1 1/2 cup full-fat coconut milk + 1 1/2 cups water)
- Stevia to taste

Directions:

1. Put the almond milk into a pitcher. Put ground cinnamon, hemp, vanilla extract in a small deep cooking pan on moderate to high heat. Heat until the pure liquid stevia is just melted and then pour the pure liquid stevia mixture into the pitcher.
2. Stir until the pure liquid stevia is well blended with the almond milk. Bring the pitcher in your refrigerator and let it cool for minimum two hours. Stir thoroughly before you serve.

Nutritional Info: Calories: 656 kcal ‖ Protein: 42.12 g ‖ Fat: 33.05 g ‖ Carbohydrates: 44.45 g

Wassail
Time To Prepare: five minutes
Time to Cook: ten minutes
Yield: Servings 4
Ingredients:

- ½ tsp nutmeg
- 1 inch peeled ginger
- 10 cloves
- 2 vanilla beans, split or 2 Tbsp pure vanilla extract
- 4 cups orange juice
- 5 cinnamon sticks
- 8 cups apple cider
- Zest and juice of 2 lemons

Directions:

1. Pour cider and orange juice in the instant pot.
2. Put cinnamon sticks, nutmeg piece, cloves, lemon zest, vanilla beans in the steamer basket.
3. If you didn't use vanilla beans, pour in vanilla extract. Put in lemon juice.

4. Secure the lid. Cook on HIGH pressure ten minutes.
5. When done, depressurize naturally.
6. Discard contents of the steamer basket.
7. Serve hot from the pot.

Nutritional Info: Calories: 221 ‖ Fat: 0g ‖ Carbohydrates: 42g ‖ Protein: 0g

White Hot Chocolate
Time To Prepare: five minutes
Time to Cook: six minutes
Yield: Servings 2
Ingredients:

- ¼ cup cocoa powder/butter
- 2 - 2½ Tbsp honey
- 2 tsp vanilla extract
- 3 cups coconut milk
- Pinch of sea salt

Directions:

1. Put in milk, cocoa powder/butter, honey, vanilla extract, and salt to the instant pot.
2. Secure the lid. Cook on LOW pressure six minutes.
3. Depressurize swiftly.
4. Use a hand blender to blend contents 25 seconds.
5. Serve hot.

Nutritional Info: Calories: 331 ‖ Fat: 14g ‖ Carbohydrates: 47g ‖ Protein: 4g

Wonderful Watermelon Drink
Time To Prepare: five minutes
Time to Cook: 0 minutes
Yield: Servings 2
Ingredients:

- 1 cup of coconut water
- 1 cup of watermelon chunks
- 1/2 cup of tart cherries

- 2 cups of frozen mixed berries
- 2 tbsp. of chia seeds

Directions:

1. Combine all ingredients in a blender or juicer then blend until pureed.
2. Serve instantly and enjoy!

Nutritional Info: Calories: 330 kcal ‖ Protein: 10.22 g ‖ Fat: 9.71 g ‖ Carbohydrates: 53.3 g

Zesty Citrus Smoothie
Time To Prepare: five minutes
Time to Cook: 0 minutes
Yield: Servings 1
Ingredients:

- 1 cup almond milk
- 1 med orange peeled, cleaned, and cut into sections
- 1 tbsp. flaxseed oil
- 2 tsp hemp protein powder
- half cup lemon juice
- Handful of ice

Directions:

1. Mix milk, lemon juice, orange, and ice in a blender.
2. Blend for a minute, move to a glass, and mix in flaxseed oil.

Nutritional Info: Calories: 427 kcal ‖ Protein: 17.5 g ‖ Fat: 28.88 g ‖ Carbohydrates: 24.96 g

Sauces And Dressings
Apple and Tomato Dipping Sauce
Time To Prepare: ten minutes
Time to Cook: 0 minutes
Yield: Servings 2-4
Ingredients:

- ¼ cup of cider vinegar

- ¼ tsp of freshly ground black pepper
- ½ tsp of sea salt
- 1 garlic clove, finely chopped
- 1 large-sized shallot, diced
- 1 tbsp. natural tomato paste
- 1 tbsp. of extra-virgin olive oil
- 1 tbsp. of maple syrup
- 1/8 tsp of ground cloves
- 3 moderate-sized apples, roughly chopped
- 3 moderate-sized tomatoes, roughly chopped

Directions:

1. Put oil into a huge deep cooking pan and heat it up on moderate heat.
2. Put in shallot and cook until light brown for approximately 2 minutes.
3. Stir in the tomato paste, garlic, salt, pepper, and cloves for approximately half a minute. Then put in in the apples, tomatoes, vinegar, and maple syrup.
4. Bring to its boiling point then decrease the heat to allow it to simmer for approximately 30 minutes. Allow to cool for twenty additional minutes before placing the mixture into your blender. Combine the mixture until the desired smoothness is achieved.
5. Keep in a mason jar or an airtight container; place in your fridge for maximum 5 days.
6. Serve it on a burger or with fries.

Nutritional Info: ‖ Calories: 142 kcal ‖ Protein: 3 g ‖ Fat: 3.46 g ‖ Carbohydrates: 26.93 g
Balsamic Vinaigrette
Time To Prepare: ten minutes
Time to Cook: 0 minutes
Yield: Servings 2-4
Ingredients:

- ¼ tsp of freshly ground black pepper
- ½ cup of extra-virgin olive oil

- ½ cup of rice vinegar
- 1 clove of freshly minced garlic
- 1 tbsp. of honey or maple syrup
- 1 tsp of sea or kosher salt
- 2 tsp of Dijon mustard

Directions:

1. Put all ingredients in a mason jar and cover firmly. Shake thoroughly until all ingredients are blended.
2. Keep in your fridge for minimum 30 minutes before you serve to keep its freshness.
3. Serve with a salad or as your meat marinate.

Nutritional Info: ‖ Calories: 147 kcal ‖ Protein: 1.85 g ‖ Fat: 13.21 g ‖ Carbohydrates: 4.02 g

Bean Potato Spread
Time To Prepare: twenty-five minutes
Time to Cook: 0 minutes
Yield: Servings 7-8
Ingredients:

- ¼ cup sesame paste
- ½ teaspoon cumin, ground
- 1 cup garbanzo beans, drained and washed
- 1 tablespoon olive oil
- 2 tablespoons lime juice
- 2 tablespoons water
- 4 cups cooked sweet potatoes, peeled and chopped
- 5 garlic cloves, minced
- A pinch of salt

Directions:

1. Throw all the ingredients into a blender and blend to make a smooth mix.
2. Move to a container.
3. Serve with carrot, celery, or veggie sticks.

Nutritional Info: Calories 156 ‖ Fat: 3g ‖ Carbohydrates: 10g ‖ Fiber: 6g ‖ Protein: 8g

Cashew Ginger Dip
Time To Prepare: *five minutes*
Time to Cook: *0 minutes*
Yield: Servings 1
Ingredients:

- ¼ cup filtered water
- ¼ teaspoon salt
- ½ teaspoon ground ginger
- 1 cup cashews, soaked in water for about twenty minutes and drained
- 1 tablespoon extra-virgin olive oil
- 1 teaspoon lemon juice
- 2 garlic cloves
- 2 teaspoons coconut aminos
- Pinch cayenne pepper

Directions:

1. In a blender or food processor, put together the cashews, garlic, water, olive oil, aminos, lemon juice, ginger, salt, and cayenne pepper.
2. Put in the mix in a container.
3. Cover and place in your fridge until chilled. You can use store it for 4-5 days in your fridge.

Nutritional Info: Calories 124 ‖ Fat: 9g ‖ Carbohydrates: 5g ‖ Fiber: 1g ‖ Protein: 3g

Creamy Avocado Dressing
Time To Prepare: *ten minutes*
Time to Cook: *0 minutes*
Yield: Servings 2-4
Ingredients:

- ½ cup of extra-virgin olive oil
- 1 clove of garlic, chopped
- 1 tsp of honey or maple syrup

- 2 small or 1 large-sized avocado, pitted and chopped
- 2 tsp of lemon or lime juice
- 3 tbsp. of chopped parsley
- 3 tbsp. of red wine vinegar
- Onion powder
- Some Kosher salt and ground black pepper

Directions:

1. Combine all ingredients into a blender, apart from the oil. As the ingredients are mixed, progressively put in the oil into the mixture. Blend until the desired smoothness is achieved or becomes liquidy.
2. Use as a vegetable or fruit salad dressing. Put in your fridge for maximum 5 days.

Nutritional Info: ‖ Calories: 300 kcal ‖ Protein: 4.09 g ‖ Fat: 27.9 g ‖ Carbohydrates: 11.41 g

Creamy Homemade Greek Dressing
Time To Prepare: ten minutes
Time to Cook: 0 minutes
Yield: Servings 2-4
Ingredients:

- ¼ cup non-dairy milk (e.g., almond, rice milk)
- ½ cup of high-quality mayonnaise, without preservatives
- ½ tsp dried basil
- ½ tsp dried oregano
- ½ tsp parsley
- ½ tsp thyme
- 1/3 cup of extra-virgin olive oil
- 1/4 cup of white wine vinegar
- 2 cloves of garlic, minced
- 2 tbsp. of lemon or lime juice
- 2 tsp of honey
- A few tablespoons of water
- Some Kosher salt and pepper

Directions:

1. Put all together ingredients in a mason jar and shake, cover firmly, and shake thoroughly. Place in your fridge for a few hours before you serve or serve instantly on your favorite vegetable or fruit salad.
2. Shake well before use. Put in your fridge for maximum 5 days.
3. You may put in a few tablespoons of water to tune the consistency as per your preference.

Nutritional Info: ‖ Calories: 474 kcal ‖ Protein: 2.08 g ‖ Fat: 50.1 g ‖ Carbohydrates: 5.31 g

Creamy Raspberry Vinaigrette
Time To Prepare: ten minutes
Time to Cook: 0 minutes
Yield: Servings 2-4
Ingredients:

- ½ cup of raspberries
- 1 tbsp. of Dijon mustard
- 1 tbsp. of Greek yogurt
- 1/3 cup of extra-virgin olive oil
- 2 tbsp. of honey or maple syrup
- 2 tbsp. of raspberry vinegar

Directions:

1. Put all together the ingredients apart from the oil into a blender, in accordance with the ordered list. Cover and blend for ten seconds, by slowly increasing the speed.
2. After 10 seconds, reduce the speed and progressively put in the oil into the mixture. Keep the speed at a stable pace until all of the oil has been poured in. Blend until blended.
3. Store in a mason jar then place in your fridge for maximum 5 days. Serve with a vegetable or fruit salad.

Nutritional Info: ‖ Calories: 151 kcal ‖ Protein: 2.22 g ‖ Fat: 9.47 g ‖ Carbohydrates: 14.65 g

Creamy Siamese Dressing
Time To Prepare: ten minutes
Time to Cook: 0 minutes

Yield: Servings 2-4
Ingredients:

- ¼ cup of non-dairy milk (e.g., almond, rice, soymilk)
- ¼ cup of unsweetened peanut sauce
- 1 cup of mayonnaise
- 1 tbsp. of honey or maple syrup
- 1 tbsps. freshly chopped cilantro
- 2 tbsp. of unsalted peanuts
- 2 tbsp. rice vinegar

Directions:

1. Put all ingredients apart from the cilantro and peanuts into a blender and blend until the desired smoothness is achieved and creamy. Next, put in in the cilantro and peanuts and pulse the blender a few times until completely crushed and well blended. Put in a mason jar and bring it in your fridge.
2. Serve with a garden salad, pasta or as a dipping sauce.

Nutritional Info: ‖ Calories: 525 kcal ‖ Protein: 18.14 g ‖ Fat: 45.55 g ‖ Carbohydrates: 11.01 g

Cucumber and Dill Sauce
Time To Prepare: ten minutes
Time to Cook: 0 minutes
Yield: Servings 2-4
Ingredients:

- ¼ cup of lemon juice
- 1 cucumber, peeled and squeezed to remove surplus liquid
- 1 cup of freshly chopped dill
- 1 tsp of sea salt
- 450g of Greek yogurt

Directions:

1. In a moderate-sized container, put together the yogurt, cucumber, and dill then stir until well blended. Put in in the lemon juice and salt to taste.

2. Cover and place in your fridge for approximately 1-2 hours before you serve to keep its freshness. Best serve with Mediterranean food, chips, fish, or even bread.

Nutritional Info: ‖ Calories: 97 kcal ‖ Protein: 13.49 g ‖ Fat: 2.1 g ‖ Carbohydrates: 6.34 g

Dairy-Free Creamy Turmeric Dressing
Time To Prepare: ten minutes
Time to Cook: 0 minutes
Yield: Servings 2-4
Ingredients:

- ½ cup of extra-virgin olive oil
- ½ cup of tahini
- 1 tbsp. of turmeric powder
- 2 tbsp. of lemon juice
- 2 tsp of honey
- Some sea salt and pepper

Directions:

1. In a container, whisk all ingredients until well blended.
2. Store in a mason jar and place in your fridge for maximum 5 days.

Nutritional Info: ‖ Calories: 328 kcal ‖ Protein: 7.3 g ‖ Fat: 29.36 g ‖ Carbohydrates: 12.43 g

Herby Raita
Time To Prepare: ten minutes
Time to Cook: 0 minutes
Yield: Servings 2-4
Ingredients:

- ¼ cup of freshly chopped mint
- ¼ tsp of freshly ground black pepper
- ½ tsp of sea salt
- 1 cup of Greek yogurt
- 1 large-sized cucumber, shredded
- 1 tsp of lemon juice

Directions:

1. Combine the cucumber with ¼ tsp of salt in a sieve and leave to drain for fifteen minutes. Shake to release any surplus liquid and move to a kitchen towel. Squeeze out as much liquid as you can using the paper towel.
2. Put the cucumber into a medium container then mix in the rest of the ingredients until well blended.
3. Put in your fridge for minimum 2 hours to keep its freshness. Best consume with spicy foods as it could relief the spiciness.

Nutritional Info: ‖ Calories: 69 kcal ‖ Protein: 4.33 g ‖ Fat: 3.66 g ‖ Carbohydrates: 4.93 g

Homemade Ginger Dressing
Time To Prepare: ten minutes
Time to Cook: 0 minutes
Yield: Servings 2-4
Ingredients:

- ¼ cup of chopped celery
- ¼ cup of honey or maple syrup
- ¼ cup of water
- ½ cup of chopped carrots
- ½ tsp of white pepper
- 1 cup of chopped onion
- 1 cup of extra-virgin olive oil
- 1 tsp of freshly minced garlic
- 1 tsp of kosher salt
- 2 ½ tbsp. of unsalted, gluten-free soy sauce
- 2 tbsp. of ketchup
- 2/3 cup of rice vinegar
- 6 tbsp. of freshly grated ginger

Directions:

1. Put the onion, ginger, celery, carrots, and garlic into a blender. Blend until the mixture are fine but still lumpy from the small vegetable chunks.
2. Put in in the vinegar, water, ketchup, soy sauce, honey or maple

syrup, lemon juice, salt, and pepper. Pulse until the ingredients are well blended.

3. Slowly put in the oil while blending, until everything is thoroughly combined. The mixture must be runny but still grainy.

4. Serve with a winter salad.

Nutritional Info: ‖ Calories: 389 kcal ‖ Protein: 2.71 g ‖ Fat: 32.08 g ‖ Carbohydrates: 22.14 g

Homemade Lemon Vinaigrette
Time To Prepare: ten minutes
Time to Cook: 0 minutes
Yield: Servings 2-4
Ingredients:

- ¼ tsp of sea salt
- ½ tsp of Dijon mustard, without preservatives
- ½ tsp of lemon zest
- 1 tsp of honey or maple syrup
- 2 tbsp. of freshly squeezed lemon juice
- 3 tbsp. of extra-virgin olive oil
- Freshly ground black pepper

Directions:

1. Whisk all together the ingredients apart from olive oil and black pepper in a small container. Then progressively put in 3 tbsp. of olive oil while continuously whisking until well blended. Put in some ground black pepper to taste.

2. Put mason jar and place in your fridge for maximum 3 days.

3. Serve with a garden salads.

Nutritional Info: ‖ Calories: 68 kcal ‖ Protein: 1.69 g ‖ Fat: 6.06 g ‖ Carbohydrates: 1.71 g

Homemade Ranch
Time To Prepare: ten minutes
Time to Cook: 0 minutes
Yield: Servings 2-4
Ingredients:

- ¼ cup of Greek yogurt
- ¼ tsp Kosher salt
- ½ cup of natural mayonnaise, without preservatives
- ½ tsp of dried dill
- ½ tsp of dried parsley
- ½ tsp of garlic powder
- ½ tsp of onion powder
- ¾ cup of non-dairy milk
- 1/8 tsp Freshly ground black pepper
- 2 tsp of dried chives

Directions:

1. Combine all ingredients apart from the milk into a medium container. Mix together until well blended.
2. Put in in the milk and mix thoroughly.
3. Pour in a mason jar or an airtight container. Serve instantly or place in your fridge for maximum 2 hours to keep the freshness. Put in your refrigerator for maximum 5 days.
4. Serve with a garden or fruit salad.

Nutritional Info: ‖ Calories: 482 kcal ‖ Protein: 3.55 g ‖ Fat: 51.98 g ‖ Carbohydrates: 1.63 g

Honey Bean Dip
Time To Prepare: five minutes
Time to Cook: 0 minutes
Yield: Servings 3-4
Ingredients:

- ¼ teaspoon ground cumin
- ¼ teaspoon salt
- 1 (14-ounce) can each of kidney beans and black beans
- 1 tablespoon apple cider vinegar
- 1 teaspoon lime juice
- 2 cherry tomatoes
- 2 garlic cloves
- 2 tablespoons filtered water
- 2 teaspoons raw honey
- Freshly ground black pepper to taste

- Pinch cayenne pepper to taste

Directions:

1. In a blender or food processor, put together the beans, garlic, tomatoes, water, vinegar, honey, lime juice, cumin, salt, cayenne pepper, and black pepper.
2. Blend until it becomes smooth. Put in the mix in a container.
3. Cover and place in your fridge to chill. You can place in your fridge for maximum 5 days.

Nutritional Info: Calories 158 ‖ Fat: 1g ‖ Carbohydrates: 33g ‖ Fiber: 8g ‖ Protein: 9g

Soy with Honey and Ginger Glaze
Time To Prepare: ten minutes
Time to Cook: 0 minutes
Yield: Servings 2-4
Ingredients:

- ¼ cup of honey
- 1 tbsp. of rice vinegar
- 1 tsp of freshly grated ginger
- 2 tbsp. gluten-free soy sauce

Directions:

1. Put all together the ingredients into a small container and whisk well.
2. Serve with a vegetables, chickens, or seafood.
3. Keep the glaze in a mason jar, firmly covered, and place in your fridge for maximum four days.

Nutritional Info: ‖ Calories: 90 kcal ‖ Protein: 2.32 g ‖ Fat: 1.54 g ‖ Carbohydrates: 17.99 g

Strawberry Poppy Seed Dressing
Time To Prepare: ten minutes
Time to Cook: 0 minutes
Yield: Servings 2-4
Ingredients:

- ¼ cup of raspberry vinegar
- ¼ tsp of ground ginger
- ¼ tsp of sea salt
- ½ tsp of onion powder
- ½ tsp of poppy seeds
- 1/3 cup of extra-virgin olive oil
- 1/3 cup of honey
- 2 tbsp. of freshly squeezed orange juice

Directions:

1. Put all ingredients, apart from the poppy seeds and oil into a blender. Blend until the desired smoothness is achieved and creamy. Next, progressively put the oil into the mixture until blended. Put in in the poppy seeds and stir thoroughly.
2. Put in a mason jar then place in your fridge before you serve. Keep for maximum 3 days.
3. Serve with your garden salads.

Nutritional Info: ‖ Calories: 167 kcal ‖ Protein: 1.84 g ‖ Fat: 9.35 g ‖ Carbohydrates: 18.89 g

Tahini Dip
Time To Prepare: ten minutes
Time to Cook: 0 minutes
Yield: Servings 2-4
Ingredients:

- ¼ cup of tahini
- ½ tsp of maple syrup
- 1 small grated or thoroughly minced clove of garlic (this is optional)
- 1 tbsp. of apple cider vinegar
- 1 tbsp. of freshly squeezed lemon juice
- 1 tbsp. of tamari
- 1 tsp of finely grated ginger, or ½ tsp of ground ginger
- 1 tsp of turmeric
- 1/3 cup of water

Directions:

1. Blend or whisk all ingredients together. Place the dressing in an airtight container then place in your fridge for approximately 5 days.
2. Enjoy!

Nutritional Info: ‖ Calories: 120 kcal ‖ Protein: 4.77 g ‖ Fat: 9.63 g ‖ Carbohydrates: 5.12 g

Tomato and Mushroom Sauce
Time To Prepare: ten minutes
Time to Cook: 0 minutes
Yield: Servings 2-4
Ingredients:

- ½ cup of water
- 1 moderate-sized leek, chopped
- 2 moderate-sized carrots, chopped
- 2 stalks of celery, chopped
- 2 tsp of dried oregano
- 4 cloves of garlic, crushed
- 450g of button mushrooms, diced
- 5 tbsp. of coconut milk
- 680g of unsalted tomato puree
- Black pepper, seasoning
- Some sea salt, seasoning

Directions:

1. In a big frying pan, place a few tablespoons of water and heat on moderate heat. Once it sizzles, put in in the mushrooms and Sautee for approximately five minutes, stir once in a while.
2. Next, put in in the leek, carrots, and celery. Stir thoroughly and cook for approximately five minutes or until the vegetables are soft. Put in more water if required.
3. Mix in the tomato puree with ½ cup of water and dried oregano. Bring to its boiling point and then decrease the heat to allow it to simmer for approximately fifteen minutes.
4. Remove from heat and mix in the garlic, coconut milk, and salt and pepper to taste.
5. Put in an airtight container, then store for maximum four days

in your fridge or freeze for maximum 1 month. Serve with a pasta.

Nutritional Info: ‖ Calories: 467 kcal ‖ Protein: 16.91 g ‖ Fat: 3.81 g ‖ Carbohydrates: 109.68 g

Snacks

Almond and Honey Homemade Bar

Time To Prepare: fifteen minutes + thirty minutes refrigerator time

Time to Cook: fifteen minutes

Yield: Servings 8

Ingredients:

- ¼ cup almond butter
- ¼ cup honey
- ¼ cup sugar (or another sweetener to your taste in adjusted amount)
- ¼ cup sunflower seeds
- ½ teaspoon vanilla extract
- 1 cup oats
- 1 cup whole-grain puffed cereal (unsweetened)
- 1 tbsp. flaxseeds
- 1 tbsp. sesame seeds
- 1/3 cup apricots (dried and chopped)
- 1/3 cup currants
- 1/3 cup raisins (chopped)
- 1/8 tsp salt
- A ¼ cup of almonds

Directions:

1. Preheat your oven to 350 degrees Fahrenheit.
2. Place a baking paper to an 8-inch pan or coat it with cooking spray/oil.
3. Combine the almonds, oats, and seeds and spread the mixture on a rimmed baking sheet.
4. Bake the mixture until you notice that the oats are mildly toasted (for approximately ten minutes).
5. Move the mixture to a container.
6. Put in cereal, raisins, currants, and apricots to the container.

7. Toss thoroughly to blend.
8. Mix honey, almond butter, vanilla, salt, and sugar in a deep cooking pan.
9. Heat on moderate heat. Stir regularly for 2-5 minutes until you see light bubbles.
10.   Once you notice the bubbles, pour the mixture over the dry mixture with apricots and oats you prepared previously.
11.   Mix thoroughly using a spatula. There mustn't be any dry spots.
12.   Move the new mixture to the previously prepared pan.
13.   Push it to the pan to make a firm and flat layer.
14.   Place in your refrigerator for half an hour
15.   Chop the layer into eight equal bars or squares, to your taste.
16.   Consume instantly or place in your refrigerator up to seven days.

Nutritional Info: ‖ Calories: 213 kcal ‖ Protein: 6.92 g ‖ Fat: 9.59 g ‖ Carbohydrates: 32.33 g

Almonds and Blueberries Yogurt Snack
Time To Prepare: ten minutes
Time to Cook: 0 minutes
Yield: Servings 2
Ingredients:

- 1 ½ cups nonfat Greek yogurt
- 1 cup blueberries
- 20 almonds, chopped

Directions:

1. Take 2 bowls and put in ¾ cup yogurt into each container.
2. Split the blueberries among the bowls and stir.
3. Drizzle half the almonds in each container before you serve.

Nutritional Info: ‖ Calories: 223 kcal ‖ Protein: 6.57 g ‖ Fat: 9.45 g ‖ Carbohydrates: 30.82 g

Anti-Inflammatory Key Lime Pie

Time To Prepare: twenty minutes + thirty-five minutes refrigerator time

Time to Cook: 0

Yield: Servings 8

Ingredients:

- ½ cup honey
- ½ cup Medjool dates, chopped and pitted
- 1 cup unsweetened shredded coconut
- 1 cup walnuts
- 1 teaspoon lime zest
- 1/4 teaspoon sea salt
- 3 firm avocados
- 3 tablespoons lime juice
- Lime slices
- Pinch of sea salt

Directions:

1. Use a food processor to put all together the walnuts, coconut, and the salt, then pulse until crudely ground.
2. Place the dates and pulse until the mixture resembles bread crumbs, trying to stick together.
3. Push the mixture into the edges and bottom of a non-stick greased 9-inch pie pan. Use your fingers or the back of a spoon to press the crust into a uniform layer. Bring the crust into the freezer for minimum fifteen minutes while preparing the filling.
4. Use the food processor again and mix the avocado, honey, lime juice, lime zest, and salt. Process until the desired smoothness is achieved.
5. Pour the filling into the now-chilled piecrust and place it in your fridge for about twenty minutes.
6. Decorate using fresh lime slices and serve cold. Store any left overs in your fridge.

Nutritional Info: ‖ Calories: 273 kcal ‖ Protein: 4.19 g ‖ Fat: 18.4 g ‖ Carbohydrates: 28.49 g

Ants on a Log

Time To Prepare: five minutes

Time to Cook: 0 minutes
Yield: Servings 2
Ingredients:

- 3 tablespoons of almond butter
- 3 tablespoons of raisins
- 6 celery sticks

Directions:

1. Spread half a tablespoon of almond butter on each celery stick.
2. Top with half a tablespoon of raisins on each celery stick.
3. Split the celery sticks between two plates, and enjoy!

Nutritional Info: ‖ Total Carbohydrates: 17g ‖ Fiber: 2g ‖ Net Carbohydrates: ‖ Protein: 4g ‖ Total Fat: 14g ‖ Calories: 201

Apple Crisp
Time To Prepare: fifteen minutes
Time to Cook: twenty-five minutes
Yield: Servings 6-8
Ingredients:
Topping:

- 1 ½ cups old-fashioned rolled oats
- 1 teaspoon salt
- ½ cup stevia
- 2 teaspoons ground cinnamon
- 1 cup nuts, crudely chopped
- 3 tablespoon melted coconut oil.
- 1/3 cup almond meal
- 2/3 cup shredded, unsweetened coconut
- 1/4 teaspoon ground nutmeg

Apple filling:

- ½ cup stevia
- 1 tablespoon ground cinnamon
- 1 teaspoon vanilla
- 1/4 cup arrowroot flour

- 1/4 teaspoon salt
- 10 tart apples
- 2 tablespoons fresh-squeezed lemon juice
- 3 tablespoons melted coconut oil
- The zest of 1 orange

Directions:

1. Set the oven to 350 F then grease a 9 by a 13-inch baking pan with coconut oil.
2. Put together the topping ingredients in a container, then mix and save for later.
3. Combine the filling ingredients (except for the apples) in a second big container.
4. Leave the skins on the apples, if you wish. Core them and slice super slim (1/8 inch thick).
5. Toss the apples in the filling ingredients to coat uniformly. Put the apple mixture in a baking pan and spread the topping over it all, pushing down tightly.
6. Put in your oven with a pan underneath to catch any drips.
7. Bake for about twenty-five minutes or until the topping is brown and juices are bubbling. Apples must be tender.
8. Cool slightly on a rack then serve.

Nutritional Info: ‖ Calories: 446 kcal ‖ Protein: 6.15 g ‖ Fat: 27.39 g ‖ Carbohydrates: 57.45 g

Apple Sauce Treat
Time To Prepare: ten minutes
Time to Cook: 0 minutes
Yield: Servings 1
Ingredients:

- ½ teaspoon cinnamon
- 1 ½ teaspoons toasted slivered almonds
- 1/4 cup low Fat cottage cheese
- 1/4 cup unsweetened applesauce

Directions:

1. Combine the cottage cheese and applesauce in a container, stirring well.
2. Drizzle with cinnamon and mix thoroughly.
3. Drizzle the top with almonds, pick up your spoon, and enjoy.

Nutritional Info: ‖ Calories: 225 kcal ‖ Protein: 16.24 g ‖ Fat: 14.17 g ‖ Carbohydrates: 8.54 g

Avocado and Egg Sandwich
Time To Prepare: ten minutes
Time to Cook: 0 minutes
Yield: Servings 2
Ingredients:

- ½ lime juice
- 1 avocado (ripe)
- 1 egg, organic
- 1 scallion
- 2 radishes
- 2 slices of who wheat, seed bread
- A pinch of salt (sea or Himalayan)
- Black pepper – to your taste
- Mixed seeds – to your choice

Directions:

1. Peel the avocado.
2. Boil the egg (soft boiled).
3. Chop the radishes to thin slices.
4. Dice the scallion (finely).
5. Mix avocado, salt, and lime juice in a container. Mash the mixture meticulously.
6. Spread the mixture onto the bread.
7. Put in some radish.
8. Put tender boiled eggs on top.
9. Put in some scallion, seeds, and pepper.

Nutritional Info: ‖ Calories: 342 kcal ‖ Protein: 12.36 g ‖ Fat: 22.99 g ‖ Carbohydrates: 26.54 g

Avocado Hummus

Time To Prepare: fifteen minutes
Time to Cook: o minutes
Yield: Servings 4
Ingredients:

- .25 cup Sunflower seeds
- .25 cup Tahini
- .25 tsp. Pepper
- .5 cup Cilantro
- .5 cup Coconut oil
- .5 Lemon juice
- .5 tsp. Salt
- 1 clove pressed garlic
- 3 Avocados
- 5 tsp. Cumin

Directions:

1. Halve the avocados, take off the pits, then spoon out the flesh.
2. Put all together ingredients in a blender and stir until super smooth.
3. Put in water, lemon juice, or oil if you need to loosen the mixture bit.

Nutritional Info: ‖ Calories: 651 kcal ‖ Protein: 9.62 g ‖ Fat: 64.05 g ‖ Carbohydrates: 19.95 g

Avocado with Tomatoes and Cucumber
Time To Prepare: ten minutes
Time to Cook: o minutes
Yield: Servings 2
Ingredients:

- ¼ cup cilantro
- ¼ cup olives – to your choice
- ½ red onion
- 1 cucumber
- 1 lemon
- 1 Tbsp. turmeric
- 1/8 cup parsley

- 2 avocados
- 4 Roma tomatoes
- Salt and pepper – to your taste

Directions:

1. Dice the tomatoes, cucumber, avocado, and olives.
2. Cut the cilantro, parsley, and onion.
3. Put in the above ingredients into a container.
4. Squeeze the lemon juice then put in to the vegetables.
5. Put in olive oil, turmeric, salt, and pepper.
6. Toss thoroughly.
7. Consume instantly after putting in lemon juice and olive oil.
8. If you prefer to consume the salad later, put in the dressing instantly before consuming it.

Nutritional Info: ‖ Calories: 480 kcal ‖ Protein: 11.57 g ‖ Fat: 35.27 g ‖ Carbohydrates: 39.77 g

Baked Veggie Turmeric Nuggets
Time To Prepare: ten minutes
Time to Cook: twenty-five minutes
Yield: Servings 24
Ingredients:

- ¼ tsp. Black pepper powder
- ¼ tsp. Sea salt
- ½ cup Almond meal
- ½ tsp. Turmeric powder
- 1 big Whole egg
- 1 cup Chopped carrots
- 1 tsp. Minced garlic
- 2 cups Broccoli florets
- 2 cups Cauliflower florets

Directions:

1. Preheat your oven to 400°F.
2. Get a parchment-lined baking sheet ready.

3. Pour cauliflower, turmeric, broccoli, carrots, black pepper, garlic, and sea salt in the blender and blitz until it's smooth.
4. Pour in the egg and almond meal and stir until it's blended.
5. Pour the paste into a mixing container. Scoop out a small amount onto your hand and make a circular disc. Put this disc on the baking sheet and repeat the pulse until the mixing container is empty.
6. Slide into the oven then bake for minimum fifteen minutes on one before flipping and baking for about ten minutes on the other side.
7. Serve with a side of Paleo ranch sauce.

Nutritional Info: ‖ Calories: 12 kcal ‖ Protein: 0.88 g ‖ Fat: 0.52 g ‖ Carbohydrates: 1.12 g

Berry Delight
Time To Prepare: fifteen minutes
Time to Cook: 0 minutes
Yield: Servings 6
Ingredients:

- ¼ cup of raw honey
- 1 cup of fresh organic blackberries
- 1 cup of fresh organic blueberries
- 1 cup of fresh organic raspberries
- 1 tablespoon of cinnamon

Directions:

1. Mix all the berries together in a big container, put in in the honey, and slowly stir.
2. Drizzle with the cinnamon.

Nutritional Info: ‖ Total Carbohydrates: 20g ‖ Fiber: 3g ‖ Net Carbohydrates: ‖ Protein: 1g ‖ Total Fat: 0g ‖ Calories: 78

Berry Energy bites
Time To Prepare: ten minutes
Time to Cook: 0 minutes
Yield: Servings 6
Ingredients:

- ¼ cup of dried blueberries
- ½ - 1 cup of almond milk
- ½ cup of coconut flour
- 1 tablespoon of coconut sugar
- 1 teaspoon of cinnamon

Directions:

1. In a huge mixing container, put together the coconut flour, cinnamon, coconut sugar, and blueberries, and mix thoroughly.
2. Put in the almond milk slowly until a firm dough is formed.
3. Form into bite-sized balls and place in your fridge for thirty minutes so they can harden up.
4. Store leftovers in your fridge.

Nutritional Info: ‖ Total Carbohydrates: 18g ‖ Fiber: 1g ‖ Net Carbohydrates: ‖ Protein: 1g ‖ Total Fat: 1g ‖ Calories: 80

Blueberry & Chia Flax Seed Pudding
Time To Prepare: ten minutes
Time to Cook: fifteen minutes
Yield: Servings 4
Ingredients:

- ¼ cup of blueberries
- 2 cups of almond milk
- 3 tablespoons of chia seeds
- 3 tablespoons of ground flaxseed

Directions:

1. Warm a pan on moderate heat then put all together of the ingredients apart from the blueberries.
2. Stir all the ingredients until the pudding is thick, this will take around three minutes.
3. Place the pudding into a container then top with blueberries.

Nutritional Info: ‖ Total Carbohydrates: 23g ‖ Fiber: 12g ‖ Net Carbohydrates: ‖ Protein: 7g ‖ Total Fat: 15g ‖ Calories: 243

Boiled Okra and Squash

Time To Prepare: five minutes
Time to Cook: five minutes
Yield: Servings 1
Ingredients:

- ½ cup of okra, cut in 1" cubes
- ½ cup of squash, cut in 1" cubes
- 1 clove garlic, minced
- 2/3 cup Vegetable stock or fish stock, plain water may be used as well
- Salt to taste

Directions:

1. Boil the liquid in high heat.
2. Put in the okra and squash. Bring to its boiling point. Put in the garlic. Reduced the heat and simmer for minimum five minutes or until the squash is soft.
3. Put in salt to taste and serve hot.

Nutritional Info: ‖ Calories: 117 kcal ‖ Protein: 8.2 g ‖ Fat: 6.25 g ‖ Carbohydrates: 7.82 g

Brownies Avocado
Time To Prepare: ten minutes
Time to Cook: twenty-five minutes
Yield: Servings 6-8
Ingredients:

- ½ cup almond meal
- 1 ½ teaspoon instant coffee (with or without caffeine, as you wish)
- 2 teaspoons ground cinnamon
- ½ teaspoon salt
- 2 cups nuts or seeds, chopped
- 1 avocado
- 1 apple, cored and chopped, with the skin on
- 1 cup cooked and diced sweet potato
- 4 tablespoons ground chia seeds
- 1 teaspoon vanilla

- ½ cup almond butter
- ½ cup coconut butter, softened
- 1/4 cup coconut oil
- 2 1/4 cup stevia
- 3/4 cup cocoa powder

Directions:

1. Set the oven to 350F then line a 9 by 13-inch pan with parchment. Allow it to overlap the sides to make handles for lifting the brownies out when done.
2. In a container, mix the almond meal, cocoa, coffee, cinnamon, salt, and nuts. Whisk and save for later.
3. Bring the remaining ingredients in a food processor and mix until the desired smoothness is achieved. Put in the ingredients in the container and pulse. This combination must be lumpy.
4. Pour into pan and bake for minimum twenty-five minutes.
5. Allow to cool and chill in your fridge for a couple of hours before cutting. The baked product will be a little gooey, so refrigerating it makes the brownies easier to cut. The chilled results will be fairly crumbly.

Nutritional Info: ‖ Calories: 591 kcal ‖ Protein: 11.03 g ‖ Fat: 53.8 g ‖ Carbohydrates: 26.58 g

Bruschetta
Time To Prepare: 60 minutes
Time to Cook: 0 minutes
Yield: Servings 4
Ingredients:

- ¼ cup of extra virgin olive oil
- ¼ teaspoon of ground black pepper
- 1 red onion, diced
- 1 teaspoon of sea salt
- 2 cloves of garlic, minced
- 2 tablespoons of balsamic vinegar
- 4 medium tomatoes, diced

Directions:

1. Put all together the ingredients into a big container, and stir slowly.
2. Place in your fridge for an hour before you serve on gluten-free toast (toast is not included in nutritional information)

Nutritional Info: ‖ Total Carbohydrates: 8g ‖ Fiber: 2g ‖ Net Carbohydrates: ‖ Protein: 1g ‖ Total Fat: 14g ‖ Calories: 156

Brussels Sprout Chips
Time To Prepare: ten minutes
Time to Cook: ten minutes
Yield: Servings 4
Ingredients:

- 2 cups Brussels sprout leaves
- 2 tablespoons ghee
- Kosher salt
- Lemon zest

Directions:

1. Set the oven to 350F, then cover two cookie sheets using parchment paper.
2. Place the leaves in a huge container and pour melted ghee over the top, and put in salt.
3. Bake for minimum 8 to ten minutes or until the leaves are crunchy. If they are tender at all, put them back in your oven.
4. While still hot, drizzle the lemon zest over the leaves. Serve warm.

Nutritional Info: ‖ Calories: 42 kcal ‖ Protein: 3.13 g ‖ Fat: 1.68 g ‖ Carbohydrates: 4.77 g

Buttered Banana Chickpea Cookies
Time To Prepare: ten minutes
Time to Cook: twelve minutes
Yield: Servings 8
Ingredients:

- ¼-tsp cinnamon
- ¼-tsp salt

- ⅓ -cup chocolate chips
- ⅓ -cup coconut sugar
- ½-cup creamy peanut butter
- 1-pc small banana, very ripe
- 1-tsp baking powder
- 2-Tbsps ground flaxseed
- 2-tsp vanilla extract
- fifteen-oz. chickpeas, washed and drained

Directions:

1. Preheat the oven to 350F. Grease a baking pan with cooking spray.
2. Mix in all the ingredients apart from the chocolate chips in your blender. Combine the batter for two minutes, or until turning into a smooth consistency.
3. Mix in the chocolate chips. Ladle the batter to make cookies. Put the cookies in the pan, and bake for about twelve minutes.

Nutritional Info: ‖ Calories: 372 ‖ Fat: 12.4g ‖ Protein: 18.6g ‖ Sodium: 174mg ‖ Total Carbohydrates: 58.1g ‖ Fiber: 11.6g ‖ Net Carbohydrates: 46.5g

Candied Dates
Time To Prepare: five minutes
Time to Cook: 0 minutes
Yield: Servings 2
Ingredients:

- 2 tablespoons of dark cocoa nibs
- 2 tablespoons of peanut butter
- 4 pitted Medjool dates

Directions:

1. Cut the pitted dates in half, and spread half a tablespoon of peanut butter on each date.
2. Top each date with half a tablespoon of dark cocoa nibs.
3. Split the candied dates between two plates, and enjoy!

Nutritional Info: ‖ Total Carbohydrates: 20g ‖ Fiber: 3g ‖ Net Carbohydrates: ‖ Protein: 5g ‖ Total Fat: 12g ‖ Calories: 187

Carrot Sticks with Avocado Dip
Time To Prepare: ten minutes
Time to Cook: 0 minutes
Yield: Servings 6
Ingredients:

- ½ cup cilantro, firmly packed
- ½ onion
- 1 big avocado, pitted
- 1 tablespoon of chili-garlic sauce or chili sauce
- 2 tablespoon olive oil
- 6 ounces shelled edamame
- Juice of one lemon
- Salt and pepper

Directions:

1. Put the edamame, cilantro, onion, and chili sauce in a blender or food processor. Pulse it to cut and mix the ingredients. Put in the avocado and the lemon juice. Slowly put in the olive oil as you blend. Move to a jar.
2. Scoop 2 spoons and serve with carrot sticks.

Nutritional Info: ‖ Calories: 154 kcal ‖ Protein: 5.16 g ‖ Fat: 11.96 g ‖ Carbohydrates: 8.44 g

Cashew "Humus"
Time To Prepare: ten minutes
Time to Cook: 0 minutes
Yield: Servings 1
Ingredients:

- ¼ Cup Water
- ¼ Teaspoon Sea Salt, Fine
- ½ Teaspoon Ground Ginger
- 1 Cup Cashews, Raw & Soaked in Water for fifteen Minutes & Drained
- 1 Tablespoon Olive Oil

- 1 Teaspoon Lemon juice, Fresh
- 2 Cloves Garlic
- 2 Teaspoon Coconut Aminos
- Pinch Cayenne Pepper

Directions:

1. Blend all ingredients together, and ensure to scrape the sides.
2. Continue to combine until the desired smoothness is achieved, and then place in your fridge it before you serve.

Nutritional Info: ‖ Calories: 112 ‖ Protein: 2.9 Grams ‖ Fat: 8.8 Grams ‖ Carbohydrates: 5.3 Grams

Cashew Cheese
Time To Prepare: 2 hours
Time to Cook: 0 minutes
Yield: Servings 6
Ingredients:

- ¼ cup of fresh basil
- 1 cup of raw cashews
- 1 tablespoon of nutritional yeast
- Juice of ½ lemon
- Salt and pepper to taste

Directions:

1. In a1 cup of water, soak the cashew for minimum 2 hours. Drain.
2. Put the cashews, lemon juice, nutritional yeast, and fresh basil into a food processor and pulse until the desired smoothness is achieved. Put in 1 tablespoon of water at a time to make it creamy, but not runny.
3. Flavor it with pepper and salt, then spread it on gluten-free bread or toast.
4. Store in an airtight jar in your fridge.

Nutritional Info: ‖ Total Carbohydrates: 126g ‖ Fiber: 1g ‖ Net Carbohydrates: ‖ Protein: 4g ‖ Total Fat: 10g ‖ Calories: 126

Cauliflower Snacks
Time To Prepare: ten minutes
Time to Cook: 60 minutes
Yield: Servings 4
Ingredients:

- 1 head of cauliflower
- 1 teaspoon salt
- 4 tablespoons extra virgin olive oil

Directions:

1. Set the oven to 425F, then prepare two cookie sheets by lining them using parchment paper.
2. Trim off the cauliflower florets and discard the core. Chop the florets into golf-ball-sized pieces.
3. Put the cauliflower in a container, and pour olive oil over them and drizzle with salt. Mix to coat. Spread in a single layer, not touching.
4. Roast approximately 1 hour flipping the cauliflower three to four times until a golden-brown color is achieved. Serve warm.

Nutritional Info: ‖ Calories: 91 kcal ‖ Protein: 2.93 g ‖ Fat: 7.7 g ‖ Carbohydrates: 3.29 g

Cereal Chia Chips
Time To Prepare: ten minutes
Time to Cook: thirty minutes
Yield: Servings 10
Ingredients:

- ¼-cup rolled oats, gluten-free
- ½-cup maple syrup
- ½-cup white quinoa, uncooked
- ¾-cup pecans, chopped
- 2-Tbsps chia seeds
- 2-Tbsps coconut oil
- 2-Tbsps coconut sugar
- A pinch of sea salt (not necessary)

Directions:

1. Preheat the oven to 325°F. Coat a baking pan using parchment paper.
2. Mix in the first six ingredients in a mixing container. Mix thoroughly until meticulously blended. Set aside.
3. Pour the oil and syrup in a small deep cooking pan placed on moderate to low heat. Heat the mixture for about three minutes, stirring once in a while.
4. Fold in the dry ingredients; stir thoroughly to coat completely.
5. Pour the mixture in the baking pan, and spread to a uniform layer using a spoon.
6. Place the pan in your oven. Bake for fifteen minutes. Turn the pan around to cook uniformly. Bake for 8-ten minutes until the mixture turns golden brown.
7. Allow cooling completely before breaking the chips into bite-size pieces.

Nutritional Info: ‖ Calories: 157 ‖ Fat: 5.2g ‖ Protein: 7.8g S ‖ Sodium: 25mg ‖ Total Carbohydrates: 22.1g ‖ Fiber: 2.5g ‖ Net Carbohydrates: 19.6g

Chewy Blackberry Leather
Time To Prepare: *fifteen minutes*
Time to Cook: *5-6 hours*
Yield: Servings 8
Ingredients:

- ¼ cup of raw honey
- 1 tbsp. of fresh mint leaves
- 1 tsp. of ground cinnamon
- 1/8 tsp. of fresh lemon juice
- 2 cups of fresh blackberries

Directions:

1. Set the oven to 170F. Coat baking sheet using parchment paper.
2. Use a food processor to put all ingredients and pulse till smooth.
3. Take the mixture onto the readied baking sheet and, using the backside of a spoon, smooth the top.

4. Bake for approximately 5-6 hours.
5. Chop the leather into equal-sized strips.
6. Now, roll each rectangle to make fruit rolls.

Nutritional Info: ‖ Calories: 49 ‖ Fat: 0.2g ‖ Carbohydrates: 12.5g ‖ Protein: 0.6g ‖ Fiber: 2.1g

Chia Cashew Cream
Time To Prepare: 2 hours and five minutes
Time to Cook: 0 minutes
Yield: Servings 1
Ingredients:

- ¼-cup quinoa, cooked
- ¼-tsp vanilla powder
- ¾-cup cashew milk
- 2-Tbsps chia seeds
- 2-Tbsps hemp hearts
- 2-Tbsps maple syrup or a dash of liquid stevia
- A pinch of cinnamon

Directions:

1. Mix all the ingredients in a jar. Mix thoroughly until meticulously blended. Cover the jar and place in your fridge for about two hours.
2. To serve, top with your desired toppings.

Nutritional Info: ‖ Calories: 258 ‖ Fat: 8.6g ‖ Protein: 12.9g ‖ Sodium: 123mg ‖ Total Carbohydrates: 34.2g ‖ Fiber: 2g ‖ Net Carbohydrates: 32.2g

Coco Cherry Bake-less Bars
Time To Prepare: ten minutes
Time to Cook: 0 minutes
Yield: Servings 6
Ingredients:

- ¼-cup pure maple syrup
- ⅓ -cup coconut, unsweetened and shredded
- ⅓ -cup dried cherries or cranberries

- ⅓ -cup ground flaxseed
- ½-cup almond butter
- 1-cup old-fashioned oats
- 1-Tbsp almond milk
- 1-Tbsp vanilla extract
- 3-scoops vanilla plant-based Protein powder

Directions:

1. Coat a loaf pan using parchment paper.
2. Mix in the first four ingredients in your blender. Blend until the mixture becomes powdery.
3. Move the mixture to a mixing container. Put in in all the rest of the ingredients. Mix thoroughly until meticulously blended.
4. Put the mixture in the pan, and press down onto a consistently flat surface.
5. Freeze for thirty minutes before cutting into six bars.

Nutritional Info: ‖ Calories: 193 ‖ Fat: 6.4g ‖ Protein: 9.6g ‖ Sodium: 200mg ‖ Total Carbohydrates: 27.1g ‖ Fiber: 3g ‖ Net Carbohydrates: 24.1g

Coconut Porridge
Time To Prepare: twenty minutes
Time to Cook: ten minutes
Yield: Servings 2
Ingredients:

- 1 tbsp. coconut oil
- 1 tsp cinnamon
- 1 vanilla bean
- 2 cups oats
- 2 tbsp. maple syrup
- 2 tsp ginger
- 2 tsp turmeric
- 330ml vaporized coconut milk
- 750 ml of water
- Coconut milk
- Fresh, shredded coconut (for serving)

Directions:

1. Mix 750 ml water and turmeric in a container. Allow it to sit for about ten minutes.
2. Combine all ingredients apart from coconut milk and shredded coconut in a deep cooking pan.
3. Heat it on medium heat while stirring continuously, and cook for eight minutes.
4. Allow it to cool for about ten minutes.
5. Split into serving bowls.
6. Put in coconut milk and shredded coconut on top.
7. Put in some extra cinnamon to your taste.
8. Eat warm.

Nutritional Info: ‖ Calories: 417 kcal ‖ Protein: 20.63 g ‖ Fat: 16.8 g ‖ Carbohydrates: 83.03 g

Cottage Cheese with Apple Sauce
Time To Prepare: five minutes
Time to Cook: 0 minutes
Yield: Servings 2
Ingredients:

- ½ teaspoon cinnamon powder
- 5-6 tablespoons cottage cheese
- two to three tablespoons applesauce or more if required

Directions:

1. Split the cottage cheese into 2 bowls.
2. Spread applesauce over the cottage cheese.
3. Drizzle ¼ teaspoon cinnamon powder on each before you serve.

Nutritional Info: ‖ Calories: 79 kcal ‖ Protein: 8.09 g ‖ Fat: 3.45 g ‖ Carbohydrates: 3.92 g

Cucumber Rolls Hors D'oeuvres
Time To Prepare: twenty minutes
Time to Cook: 0 minutes
Yield: Servings 8-10
Ingredients:

- ¼ cup fresh dill, finely chopped

- ½ cup capers
- ½ cup fresh parsley + extra to decorate, finely chopped
- 1 teaspoon Himalayan pink salt
- 2 big organic English cucumbers or 4 normal cucumbers
- 5-6 ripe avocadoes, peeled, pitted, mashed
- For the avocado spread:
- Freshly cracked pepper to taste

Directions:

1. Peel the cucumbers and cut thin slices along the length on a mandolin slicer.
2. Put the cucumber slices on your countertop.
3. To make the avocado spread: Put in all the ingredients of avocado spread into a container and stir until well blended.
4. Spread the avocado mixture uniformly and thinly on the cucumber slices.
5. Begin rolling from one of the shorter ends to the other end and place on a serving platter with its seam side facing down.
6. Repeat the above step with the rest of the cucumber slices.
7. Serve instantly as the cucumbers tend to get soggy after a while.

Nutritional Info: ‖ Calories: 227 kcal ‖ Protein: 3.77 g ‖ Fat: 19.88 g ‖ Carbohydrates: 12.99 g

Cucumber Yogurt
Time To Prepare: five minutes
Time to Cook: 0 minutes
Yield: Servings 1
Ingredients:

- 1 cup cucumbers, skin removed and chopped in chunks
- 1 teaspoon fresh dill, chopped fine
- 1/4 cup fat-free Greek yogurt
- 2 tablespoons chopped cashews
- 2 teaspoons fresh-squeezed lemon juice

Directions:

1. Peel and cut the cucumbers, then put them in a container.

2. Put in the cashews, yogurt, lemon juice, and dill.
3. Mix thoroughly, grab a spoon, and enjoy.

Nutritional Info: ‖ Calories: 300 kcal ‖ Protein: 11.35 g ‖ Fat: 23.55 g ‖ Carbohydrates: 14.13 g

Delectable Cookies
Time To Prepare: twenty minutes
Time to Cook: fifteen-twenty minutes
Yield: Servings 6
Ingredients:

- 1 cup of almonds
- ¼ cup of arrowroot flour
- 1 tbsp. of coconut flour
- 1 tsp. ground turmeric
- Salt, to taste
- Freshly ground black pepper, to taste
- 1 organic egg
- ¼ cup of olive oil
- 3 tbsp. of raw honey
- 1 tsp. of organic vanilla extract
- 1 1/3 cups of almond flour

Directions:

1. Use a food processor to put the almonds and pulse till chopped roughly
2. Move the chopped almonds in a big container.
3. Place the flours and spices and mix thoroughly.
4. In another container, put the rest of the ingredients then beat till well blended.
5. Put the flour mixture into the egg mixture and mix till well blended.
6. Position a plastic wrap over the cutting board.
7. Put the dough over the cutting board.
8. Use your hands to pat into approximately 1-inch thick circle.
9. Gently chop the circle in 6 wedges.
10. Set the scones onto a cookie sheet in a single layer.
11. Bake for approximately fifteen-20 minutes.

Nutritional Info: ‖ Calories: 335 ‖ Fat: 27.7g ‖ Carbohydrates: 17.6g ‖ Protein: 9g ‖ Fiber: 4.8g

Dried Dates & Turmeric Truffles
Time To Prepare: fifteen minutes
Time to Cook: 0 minutes
Yield: Servings 4
Ingredients:

- ¼-tsp black pepper
- ⅓ -cup walnuts
- ½-cup rolled oats
- ¾-cup dates, pitted
- 1-Tbsp turmeric powder + more for rolling

Directions:

1. Mix in all the ingredients, excluding the dates in a food processor. Blend until meticulously blended.
2. Put in the dates progressively until forming into the dough.
3. Shape and roll balls from the mixture. Roll each ball with the additional turmeric powder until coating fully.
4. Store the truffles in an airtight jar until ready to serve.

Nutritional Info: ‖ Calories: 95 ‖ Fat: 3.1g ‖ Protein: 4.7g ‖ Sodium: 62mg ‖ Total Carbohydrates: 13.8g ‖ Fiber: 2g ‖ Net Carbohydrates: 11.8g

Easy Guacamole
Time To Prepare: ten minutes
Time to Cook: 0 minutes
Yield: Servings 3
Ingredients:

- ½ Teaspoon Sea Salt
- 1 Teaspoon Garlic Powder
- 4 Avocados, Halved & Pitted

Directions:

1. Scoop your avocado flesh out, placing it in a container.

2. Put in in your salt and garlic powder mashing until it's creamy. You can place in your fridge it, and it'll keep for two days.

Nutritional Info: ‖ Calories: 358 ‖ Protein: 7.3 Grams ‖ Fat: 32.2 Grams ‖ Carbohydrates: 13.7 Grams

Easy Peasy Ginger Date
Time To Prepare: twenty minutes
Time to Cook: ten minutes
Yield: Servings 8
Ingredients:

- ¼ cup Almond milk
- ¾ cup Dates
- 1 or 1 ½ cup Almonds or almond flour
- 1 tsp. Ground ginger

Directions:

1. Preheat your oven to 350°F.
2. If you're using fresh almonds, put it through a blender to turn it to almond flour. Blitz for a couple of minutes or so until it looks and feels smooth.
3. Do not blitz for too long, or you might end up making nut butter. Now that you have your almond powder put it in a container and set it aside.
4. Pour the dates and almond milk into your blender and pulse for five minutes. If it doesn't resemble a paste, pulse for another two minutes.
5. Pour in the ground ginger and almond flour. Pulse for three to four minutes to combine.
6. Place the mixture to a baking dish and bake for approximately twenty minutes.
7. Take out of the oven and leave to cool before cutting into bits.
8. Serve or store.

Nutritional Info: ‖ Calories: 55 kcal ‖ Protein: 1.24 g ‖ Fat: 0.99 g ‖ Carbohydrates: 11.24 g

Energetic Oat Bars
Time To Prepare: ten minutes

Time to Cook: twenty-five minutes
Yield: Servings 6
Ingredients:

- ½ cup of gluten-free rolled oats
- ¾ cup fresh blueberries
- 1 peeled and mashed banana
- 1 tbsp. of chopped walnuts
- 1 tbsp. of fresh pomegranate juice
- 1 tbsp. of sunflower seeds
- 2 tbsp. of flax seeds
- 2 tbsp. of pitted and chopped finely dates
- 2 tbsp. of raisins

Directions:

1. Set the oven to 350F. Lightly, oil an 8-inch baking dish.
2. In a huge mixing container, put all ingredients and mix till well blended.
3. Put the mixture into the readied baking dish uniformly.
4. Bake for approximately twenty-five minutes. Remove from the oven then cool.
5. Using a knife, split the bars into the size your desired pieces then serve.

Nutritional Info: ‖ Calories: 88 ‖ Fat: 2.3g ‖ Carbohydrates: 18.2g ‖ Protein: 2.3g ‖ Fiber: 2.8g

Energy Dates Balls
Time To Prepare: ten minutes
Time to Cook: twenty-five minutes
Yield: Servings 7
Ingredients:

- ¼ cup of fresh lemon juice
- ½ cup of shredded sweetened coconut
- 1 cup of pitted and chopped dates
- 1 cup of toasted almonds

Directions:

1. Coat a big baking sheet using a parchment paper. Keep aside.
2. Use a food processor to add almonds and pulse till chopped crudely.
3. Put in dates and lemon juice and pulse till a tender dough forms.
4. Make equal sized balls from the mixture.
5. In a shallow, dish place shredded coconut.
6. Roll the balls in shredded coconut uniformly.
7. Place the balls onto the baking sheet in a single layer.
8. Place in your fridge to set completely before you serve.

Nutritional Info: ‖ Calories: 173 ‖ Fat: 7.9g ‖ Carbohydrates: 23g ‖ Protein: 3.8g ‖ Fiber: 4.3g

Flavorsome Almonds
Time To Prepare: ten minutes
Time to Cook: fifteen minutes
Yield: Servings 8
Ingredients:

- ¼ tsp. of cayenne pepper
- ¼ tsp. of ground cumin
- ½ tsp. of chili powder
- ½ tsp. of ground cinnamon
- 1 tbsp. of filtered water
- 1 tsp. of extra-virgin olive oil
- 2 cups of whole almonds
- 3 tbsp. of raw honey
- Salt, to taste

Directions:

1. Preheat your oven to 350 degrees F.
2. Position the almonds onto a big rimmed baking sheet in a single layer.
3. Roast for approximately ten minutes.
4. In the meantime, in a microwave-safe container, put in honey and microwave on Hugh for approximately half a minute.
5. Remove from microwave and mix in oil and water.
6. In a small container, combine all spices.

7. Take away the almonds from the oven, put in it into the container of honey mixture, and stir until blended well.

8. Move the almond mixture onto the baking sheet in a single layer.

9. Drizzle with spice mixture uniformly.

10.   Roast for approximately 3-4 minutes.

11.   Take off from oven and keep aside to cool to room temperature and serve.

12.   You can preserve these roasted almonds in an airtight jar.

Nutritional Info: ‖ Calories: 168 ‖ Fat: 12.5g ‖ Carbohydrates: 11.8g ‖ Protein: 5.1g ‖ Fiber: 3.1g

Flourless & Flaky Muffin Munchies
Time To Prepare: twenty-five minutes
Time to Cook: twenty minutes
Yield: Servings 4
Ingredients:

- ⅛-tsp baking soda
- ¼-cup peanut butter or allergy-friendly substitution
- ¼-cup pure maple syrup or honey
- ¼-tsp salt
- ½-cup quick oats or quinoa flakes, loosely packed
- ¾-tsp baking powder
- 1-cup white beans, cooked
- 1-pc medium mashed banana, very ripe
- 2-tsp pure vanilla extract
- A handful of mini chocolate chips, crushed walnuts, shredded coconut, pinch cinnamon, etc. (not necessary)

Directions:

1. Preheat your oven to 350 F. Coat 8-muffin cups with glassine.
2. Mix all the ingredients in your blender. Blend to a smooth consistency. Pour the mixture into the muffin cups at ⅔ full.
3. Place the cups in your oven, and bake for about twenty minutes.
4. Allow the muffins to sit and cool for about twenty minutes.

Nutritional Info: ‖ Calories: 119 ‖ Fat: 3.9g ‖ Protein: 8.9g ‖ Sodium: 102mg ‖ Total Carbohydrates: 14.4g ‖ Fiber: 2.5g ‖ Net Carbohydrates: 11.9g

Ginger Flour Banana Ginger Bars
Time To Prepare: ten minutes
Time to Cook: forty minutes
Yield: Servings 4-6
Ingredients:

- 1 ½ tbsp. Grated ginger
- 1 cup Coconut flour
- 1 tsp. Baking soda
- 1 tsp. Ground cardamom
- 1/3 cup Honey or maple syrup
- 1/3 cup melted butter
- 2 big Ripe bananas
- 2 tsp. Apple cider vinegar
- 2 tsp. Cinnamon
- 6 medium While eggs

Directions:

1. Preheat your oven to 350°F.
2. Coat a glass baking dish using parchment paper. If you do not have any paper, just grease the pan.
3. Put all the ingredients apart from the baking soda and apple cider vinegar through a food processor and pulse until it's all mixed up.
4. Now put in the last two ingredients and blitz once before pouring the mix into the glass dish.
5. Bake up to a toothpick inserted into the center comes out clean. This usually takes forty minutes.

Nutritional Info: ‖ Calories: 1407 kcal ‖ Protein: 42.18 g ‖ Fat: 100.26 g ‖ Carbohydrates: 88.33 g

Ginger Turmeric ‖ *Protein: Bars*
Time To Prepare: ten minutes + 20 cooling time
Time to Cook: twenty-five minutes
Yield: Servings 7

Ingredients:

- ½ cup coconut
- 1 cup cashews
- 1 scoop turmeric Protein bone broth
- 1 Tbsp. ginger
- 1/3 cup sunflower butter
- 2 Tbsp. maple syrup

Directions:

1. Put in coconut pieces and cashews to a blender or food processor. Use the pulse option to obtain a coarse mixture.
2. Put in butter, broth, maple syrup, and ginger and pulse the mixture to make a coarse, yet even and fairly sticky mass.
3. Evenly put the mixture to a baking pan (8x8 inches) with your hands or a spoon. Push tightly to the baking pan.
4. Bring it in a fridge and allow it to cool for about twenty minutes.
5. Chop the mixture into even squares.
6. You can consume instantly or store in a glass container in the refrigerator (up to 7 days).

Nutritional Info: 107 kcal ‖ Protein: 1.15 g ‖ Fat: 9.59 g ‖ Carbohydrates: 4.63 g

Hummus Deviled Eggs
Time To Prepare: ten minutes
Time to Cook: 0 minutes
Yield: Servings 6
Ingredients:

- ½ cup hummus
- 6 hard-boiled eggs
- Paprika

Directions:

1. Cut the hardboiled eggs in half along the length and remove the yolk.

2. Fill the egg whites with hummus and drizzle with paprika before you serve.

Nutritional Info: ‖ Calories: 179 kcal ‖ Protein: 11.03 g ‖ Fat: 12.41 g ‖ Carbohydrates: 5.14 g

Hummus with Celery
Time To Prepare: fifteen minutes
Time to Cook: o minutes
Yield: Servings 4
Ingredients:

- 3 cloves of garlic, crushed
- 2 tablespoons extra virgin olive oil
- ½ teaspoon salt
- ½ teaspoon cumin
- 1 (fifteen–ounce) can chickpeas
- two to three tablespoons water
- Dash of paprika
- 6 stalks celery, cut into two-inch pieces
- 3 tablespoons salsa
- 1/4 cup lemon juice
- 1/4 cup tahini

Directions:

1. Using a food processor mix the lemon juice and tahini for approximately one minute, until it is smooth. Scrape the sides down and process for 30 more seconds.
2. Put in the garlic, olive oil, salt, and cumin. Blend for approximately one minute.
3. Drain the chickpeas, put the half of them on the food processor, and blend for one more minute. Scrape down the sides, put in the other half of the chickpeas, and pulse until smooth, approximately 2 minutes. If it like a little too thick, put in water, 1 tablespoon at a time until you reach the desired consistency.
4. Fill the celery sticks with hummus and drizzle paprika on top.
5. Serve with salsa for dipping.

Nutritional Info: ‖ Calories: 240 kcal ‖ Protein: 9.27 g ‖ Fat: 14.51 g ‖ Carbohydrates: 21.01 g

Kale Chips
Time To Prepare: ten minutes
Time to Cook: 2 hours
Yield: Servings 8
Ingredients:

- ½ teaspoon sea salt
- 1 cup cashews, soaked and softened in water about 2 hours
- 1 cup grated sweet potato
- 2 bunches of curly kale with stems removed, washed and torn into bite-sized pieces
- 2 tablespoons honey
- 2 tablespoons nutritional yeast (found at health food stores)
- 2 tablespoons water
- The juice of 1 lemon

Directions:

1. Place the kale in a huge container and save for later.
2. In a blender or food processor, process the sweet potato, softened cashews yeast, lemon juice, honey, salt, and water until the desired smoothness is achieved. Place the mixture on the kale and toss with your hands to coat the leaves.
3. Spread the kale leaves out on a big cookie sheet in a single cover without touching.
4. Set the oven to its lowest setting.
5. Prop the oven door slightly ajar and dehydrate the chips for approximately 2 hours flipping the cookie sheet and watching to ensure the chips do not burn.
6. When crunchy, take it out of the oven and allow to cool. Store in an airtight container.

Nutritional Info: ‖ Calories: 40 kcal ‖ Protein: 2.19 g ‖ Fat: 0.87 g ‖ Carbohydrates: 6.39 g

Lemony Ginger Cookies
Time To Prepare: fifteen minutes + thirty minutes chill time
Time to Cook: 10-twelve minutes

Yield: Servings 25
Ingredients:

- ½ cup arrowroot flour
- ½ teaspoon baking soda
- 1 ½ cup coconut butter, softened
- 1 ½ cups stevia
- 1 teaspoon nutritional yeast
- 2 teaspoons vanilla
- 3 inches of ginger root, peeled and diced
- 3/4 teaspoon salt
- Zest of 1 lemon

Directions:

1. Set the oven to 350F, then line two or three cookie sheets using parchment paper.
2. Combine the arrowroot flour, stevia, salt, soda, and yeast in a container.
3. In another container, put the rest of the ingredients and mix thoroughly.
4. Put in the dry ingredients progressively until well blended. If the dough is too soft, put an additional one to 2 tablespoons of arrowroot powder. The dough will stiffen when chilled, so be careful.
5. Cover the dough in parchment and push it flat. Chill for half an hour
6. Take a chunk of the chilled dough and flatten it between two pieces of parchment until it is 1/8 inch thick. Sprinkle with a little arrowroot powder and slice into shapes.
7. Put on baking sheets approximately 1 inch apart and bake ten to twelve minutes. Cool on cookie sheets for fifteen minutes before removing.

Nutritional Info: ‖ Calories: 112 kcal ‖ Protein: 0.44 g ‖ Fat: 11.3 g ‖ Carbohydrates: 2.49 g

Low Cholesterol-Low Calorie Blueberry Muffin
Time To Prepare: ten minutes
Time to Cook: twenty-five minutes

Yield: Servings 12
Ingredients:

- ½ cup skim milk or non-fat milk
- ½ cup white sugar
- 1 and ½ cup of flour, all-purpose
- 1 cup blueberries, fresh
- 1 egg white
- 1 tablespoon coconut oil
- 2 tablespoons melted margarine
- 2 teaspoons baking powder
- Pinch of salt

Directions:

1. Set the oven to 205C.
2. Grease a 12-cup muffin pan using oil.
3. In a small container, put the blueberries. Put in ¼ cup of the flour and mix it together. Set aside.
4. In another container, whisk the egg white and the coconut oil. Put in the melted margarine.
5. In a different container, mix all together the dry ingredients and sift. Sift again over the egg white mixture. Mix to moisten the flour. The flour should look lumpy, so do not overmix.
6. Fold in the blueberries. Separate the blueberries, so that each scoop will have blueberries. Scoop the mixture into the muffin pans. Fill only up to two-thirds of the pan.
7. Bake for about twenty-five minutes or until the muffin turns golden brown.

Nutritional Info: ‖ Calories: 114 kcal ‖ Protein: 2.66 g ‖ Fat: 5.34 g ‖ Carbohydrates: 14.25 g

Mandarin Cottage Cheese
Time To Prepare: *five minutes*
Time to Cook: *0 minutes*
Yield: Servings 1
Ingredients:

- ½ cup canned mandarin oranges

- ½ cup low-fat cottage cheese
- 1 ½ tablespoons slivered almonds

Directions:

1. Put the cottage cheese in a container.
2. Drain the mandarin oranges, put them atop the cottage cheese, and drizzle with almonds.

Nutritional Info: ‖ Calories: 360 kcal ‖ Protein: 26.24 g ‖ Fat: 21.37 g ‖ Carbohydrates: 15.22 g

Mini Pepper Nachos
Time To Prepare: five minutes
Time to Cook: ten minutes
Yield: Servings 8
Ingredients:

- .25 tsp. Red pepper flakes
- .5 cup Tomato, chopped
- .5 tsp. Oregano
- 1 tbsp. Chili powder
- 1 tsp. Cumin, ground
- 1 tsp. Garlic powder
- 1 tsp. Paprika
- 16 oz. Ground beef
- 16 oz. Mini peppers, seeded, halved
- 5 tsp. Pepper
- 5 tsp. Salt
- cup Cheddar cheese, shredded

Directions:

1. Mix seasonings together in a container.
2. On moderate heat, brown the meat, be sure all the clumps are broken up.
3. Stir in the spices and continue to sauté until the seasoning has gone through all of the meat.
4. Heat the oven to 400F.
5. Put the peppers in a single line. They can touch.

6. Coat with the beef mix.
7. Drizzle with cheese.
8. Bake for minimum ten minutes or until cheese has melted.
9. Pull out of the oven and top with the toppings.

Nutritional Info: ‖ Calories: 240 kcal ‖ Protein: 11.01 g ‖ Fat: 18.2 g ‖ Carbohydrates: 9.49 g

Mushroom Chips
Time To Prepare: ten minutes
Time to Cook: 45-60 minutes
Yield: Servings 2-4
Ingredients:

- 16 ounces of king oyster mushrooms
- 2 tablespoons ghee
- Kosher salt and ground pepper to taste

Directions:

1. Set the oven to 300F, then line two cookie sheets using parchment paper.
2. Cut every mushroom in half along the length, then cut with a mandolin into 1/8 inch slices or strips. Put them on cookie sheets with some room in between. Melt the ghee and brush it over the mushrooms, then flavor with the salt and pepper.
3. Bake for minimum 45 minutes to an hour, until they are completely crunchy. Store in airtight containers.

Nutritional Info: ‖ Calories: 62 kcal ‖ Protein: 5.58 g ‖ Fat: 2 g ‖ Carbohydrates: 7.97 g

Olive and Tomato Balls
Time To Prepare: ten minutes
Time to Cook: thirty-five minutes
Yield: Servings 5
Ingredients:

- .25 cup Coconut oil
- .25 tsp. Salt
- .5 cup Cream cheese

- 2 cloves Garlic, crushed
- 2 tbsp. Basil, chopped
- 2 tbsp. Oregano, chopped
- 2 tbsp. Thyme, chopped
- 4 Kalamata olives, pitted
- 4 pcs. Sun-dried tomatoes, drained
- 5 tbsp. Parmesan cheese, grated
- Black pepper (as you wish)

Directions:

1. Cut the coconut oil, put in it to a small mixing container with the cream cheese, and allow them to tenderize for approximately 30 minutes. Mash together and mix thoroughly to blend.
2. Put in in the Kalamata olives and sun-dried tomatoes and mix thoroughly before you put in in the herbs and seasonings. Mix meticulously before placing the mixing container in your fridge to allow the results to solidify.
3. Once it has solidified, make the mixture into a total of 5 balls using an ice cream scoop. Roll each of the finished balls into the parmesan cheese before plating.
4. Stored the extra's in your refrigerator in an air-tight container for maximum 7 days.

Nutritional Info: ‖ Calories: 212 kcal ‖ Protein: 4.77 g ‖ Fat: 20.75 g ‖ Carbohydrates: 3.13 g

Oven Crisp Sweet Potato
Time To Prepare: ten minutes
Time to Cook: twenty minutes
Yield: Servings 2
Ingredients:

- 1 moderate-sized sweet potato, raw
- 1 teaspoon coconut oil
- 1 teaspoon sugar

Directions:

1. Preheat your oven to 160C.
2. Using a mandolin slicer or a peeler, slice the sweet potato into thin chips or strips. Rinse and pat dry.
3. Sprinkle the coconut oil over the potatoes. Toss until all chips are coated.
4. Position in an oven baking sheet. Bake for about ten minutes. Check the crispiness. If it is not that crunchy enough, bake for an extra five or 10 minutes or until the chips attain the crispiness desired.
5. Take out the crunchy sweet potatoes. Drizzle with sugar before you serve.

Nutritional Info: ‖ Calories: 123 kcal ‖ Protein: 4.23 g ‖ Fat: 5.39 g ‖ Carbohydrates: 14.63 g

Paleo Ginger Spiced Mixed Nuts
Time To Prepare: *five minutes*
Time to Cook: forty minutes
Yield: Servings 8
Ingredients:

- ½ tsp. Fine sea salt
- ½ tsp. Vietnamese cinnamon
- 1 tsp. Grated fresh ginger
- 2 cups Mix nuts; Cashew, goji berries, raw almonds, pumpkin seeds, etc.
- 2 Large Egg,
- Coconut oil spray
- Egg whites

Directions:

1. Prepare the oven by preheating to 250°F.
2. Whisk egg whites in a container until it gets fluffy. Pour in sea salt, grated ginger, and Vietnamese cinnamon. Whisk until it's one big mix.
3. Pour in the mixed nuts and stir to combine.
4. Coat the parchment-lined baking sheet with coconut oil spray and spread the nut mixture all across the baking sheet.

5. Allow it to bake for approximately twenty minutes, rotate the sheet then bake for another twenty minutes.
6. Take off the baking sheet from the oven and leave to cool.
7. Once it's fully cool and hard, break them into bits with clean hands.
8. Serve or store.

Nutritional Info: ‖ Calories: 212 kcal ‖ Protein: 6.92 g ‖ Fat: 17.3 g ‖ Carbohydrates: 10.05 g

Party-Time Chicken Nuggets
Time To Prepare: ten minutes
Time to Cook: twenty-five minutes
Yield: Servings 6
Ingredients:

- ½ cup tapioca flour
- ½ tsp. of garlic powder
- ½ tsp. of onion powder
- ½ tsp. of paprika
- 1½ cups of blanched almond flour
- 2 (6-ounce) grass-fed skinless, boneless chicken breasts
- 2 big organic eggs
- Freshly ground black pepper, to taste
- Salt, to taste

Directions:

1. Set the oven to 400F then grease a big baking sheet.
2. With a rolling pin, roll the chicken breasts to a uniform thickness.
3. Cut each breast into bite-sized pieces.
4. In a shallow dish, crack the eggs and beat thoroughly.
5. In another shallow dish, combine flours and spices.
6. Immerse the chicken nuggets in beaten eggs.
7. Then roll in flour mixture completely.
8. Position the nuggets onto the readied baking sheet in a single layer.
9. Bake for approximately 10-twelve minutes, turning once after five minutes.

Nutritional Info: ‖ Calories: 312 ‖ Fat: 17.8g ‖ Carbohydrates: 15.4g ‖ Protein: 23.6g ‖ Fiber: 3.2g

Peanut Butter and Honey Oat Bars
Time To Prepare: ten minutes
Time to Cook: twenty-five minutes
Yield: Servings 18
Ingredients:

- ¼ cup honey
- ¼ cup honey roasted peanuts, chopped
- ¼ teaspoon cinnamon powder
- ¼ teaspoon vanilla extract
- 1 cup oats
- 2 teaspoons coconut oil
- 3 tablespoons peanut butter

Directions:

1. Coat a small baking pan using a parchment paper such that the parchment paper is hanging over the sides of the baking pan.
2. Put in honey, oil, and peanut butter into a microwave-safe container. Microwave on High for around 20 -half a minute or until the peanut butter melts completely. If it takes longer than half a minute, stir and cook in increments of 10 seconds, stirring every time.
3. Remove from the microwave and put in the remaining ingredients. Mix thoroughly and pour into the readied baking pan. Spread the mixture and press using a spatula.
4. Bake in a preheated oven 300° F for approximately twenty minutes or until the top is light brown.
5. Take out of the oven and press once once more.
6. Cool for a while and slice.
7. Cool thoroughly before you serve.
8. Move leftover bars into an airtight container. Place in your fridge until use.

Nutritional Info: ‖ Calories: 44 kcal ‖ Protein: 1.47 g ‖ Fat: 1.69 g ‖ Carbohydrates: 8.06 g

Protein-Packed Croquettes

Time To Prepare: ten minutes
Time to Cook: five minutes
Yield: Servings 12
Ingredients:

- ¼ cup of chopped fresh cilantro leaves
- ¼ cup plus 1 tbsp. of olive oil, divided
- ¼ tsp. of ground turmeric
- ½ cup of thawed frozen peas
- ½ tsp. of paprika
- 1 cup of cooked quinoa
- 2 big peeled and mashed boiled potatoes
- 2 minced garlic cloves
- 2 tsp. of ground cumin
- Freshly ground black pepper, to taste
- Salt, to taste

Directions:

1. In a frying pan, heat 1 tbsp. of oil on moderate heat.
2. Put in peas and garlic and sauté for approximately one minute.
3. Move the peas mixture into a big container.
4. Put rest of the ingredients then mix till well blended.
5. Make equal sized oblong shaped patties from the mixture.
6. In a huge frying pan, warm remaining oil on moderate to high heat.
7. Put in croquettes in batches and fry for approximately 4 minutes per side.

Nutritional Info: ‖ Calories: 152 ‖ Fat: 6.9g ‖ Carbohydrates: 20.1g ‖ Protein: 3.5g ‖ Fiber: 2.9g

Roasted Beets
Time To Prepare: ten minutes
Time to Cook: 35-45 minutes
Yield: Servings 6
Ingredients:

- 1 tablespoon of coconut oil, melted
- 1 teaspoon of salt

- 2 and a ½ pounds of beets, peeled and diced

Directions:

1. Preheat your oven to 400°F.
2. Spread the beets onto a baking sheet and sprinkle with melted coconut oil.
3. Put in salt and mix thoroughly.
4. Roast the beets in your oven for 35-45 minutes, until the beets are tender.

Nutritional Info: ‖ Total Carbohydrates: 7g ‖ Fiber: 2g ‖ Net Carbohydrates: ‖ Protein: 1g ‖ Total Fat: 4g ‖ Calories: 59

Roasted Garlic Chickpeas
Time To Prepare: *five minutes*
Time to Cook: twenty minutes
Yield: Servings 2
Ingredients:

- 1 Teaspoon Garlic Powder
- 1 Teaspoon Sea Salt
- 2 Tablespoons Olive Oil
- 4 Cups Cooked Chickpeas, Rinsed, Drained & Dried
- Black Pepper to Taste

Directions:

1. Begin by heating the oven to 400.
2. Spread your chickpeas on a baking sheet, coating them with your olive oil.
3. Bake of 20 minutes, ensuring to stir them at the ten-minute mark.
4. Put your hot chickpeas in a container, seasoning before securing them in an airtight container. They'll keep at room temperature for maximum two days.

Nutritional Info: ‖ Calories: 150 ‖ Protein: 6 Grams ‖ Fat: 5 Grams ‖ Carbohydrates: 21 Grams

Salmon & Avocado Toast

Time To Prepare: ten minutes
Time to Cook: five minutes
Yield: Servings 1
Ingredients:

- ¼ tsp red pepper
- ½ avocado
- 1 tsp lemon juice
- 2 slices of gluten-free bread
- oz. pink salmon (wild)
- salt and pepper - to taste

Directions:

1. Cut the avocado.
2. Toast the bread to your taste.
3. Combine the salmon and lemon juice.
4. When the toast is ready, lay avocado slices onto it.
5. Cover with salmon.
6. Put in some red pepper, salt, and pepper to your taste.
7. Feel free to put the other ingredients you prefer (tomatoes, onions)
8. Enjoy your salmon snack!

Nutritional Info: ‖ Calories: 481 kcal ‖ Protein: 28.08 g ‖ Fat: 27.52 g ‖ Carbohydrates: 33 g

Salt & Vinegar Kale Crisps
Time To Prepare: five minutes
Time to Cook: 20-twenty-five minutes
Yield: Servings 2
Ingredients:

- 1 Teaspoon Sea Salt, Fine
- 2 Tablespoon Apple Cider Vinegar
- 2 Tablespoons Olive Oil
- 4 Cups Kale, Torn into 2 Inch Pieces

Directions:

1. Begin by heating the oven to 350. Get out a container, and mix all of your ingredients.
2. Put your kale on a baking sheet, baking for twenty to twenty-five minutes. Toss midway through this time.
3. Put at room temperature in an airtight container. They'll keep for two days.

Nutritional Info: ‖ Calories: 135 ‖ Protein: 1 Gram ‖ Fat: 14 Grams ‖ Carbohydrates: 3 Grams

Soft Flourless Cookies
Time To Prepare: ten minutes
Time to Cook: twenty-five minutes
Yield: Servings 4
Ingredients:

- ¼ teaspoon of organic vanilla extract
- ¾ cup of shredded unsweetened coconut
- 1 peeled big banana
- Pinch of ground cinnamon

Directions:

1. Set the oven to 350F. Coat a cookie sheet with a big greased parchment paper.
2. In a big food processor, put all ingredients and pulse till well blended.
3. Ladle the mixture onto the prepared cookie sheet. Use your hands to flatten the cookies slightly.
4. Bake for minimum twenty-five minutes or till golden brown.

Nutritional Info: ‖ Calories: 84 ‖ Fat: 5.1g ‖ Carbohydrates: 10.1g ‖ Protein: 0.9g ‖ Fiber: 2.3g

Spiced Nuts
Time To Prepare: ten minutes
Time to Cook: 10-fifteen minutes
Yield: Servings 2
Ingredients:

- ¼ Cup Pumpkin Puree

- ¼ Cup Sunflower Seeds
- ¼ Teaspoon Garlic Powder
- ¼ Teaspoon Red Pepper Flakes
- ½ Cup Walnuts
- ½ Teaspoon Ground Cumin
- 1 Cup Almonds
- 1 Teaspoon Ground Turmeric

Directions:

1. Begin by heating the oven to 350.
2. Mix all ingredients together, and then get out a baking sheet. Spread your nuts over your baking sheet, cooking for ten to fifteen minutes.
3. Allow it to cool well before you store it.

Nutritional Info: ‖ Calories: 180 ‖ Protein: 6 Grams ‖ Fat: 16 Grams ‖ Carbohydrates: 7 Grams

Spicy Bean Dip
Time To Prepare: ten minutes
Time to Cook: 0 minutes
Yield: Servings 3
Ingredients:

- ¼ Teaspoon Ground Cumin
- ¼ Teaspoon Sea Salt
- 1 Tablespoon Apple Cider Vinegar
- 1 Teaspoon Lime Juice, Fresh
- 14 Ounce Can Black Beans, Drained & Rinsed
- 14 Ounce Can Kidney Beans, Drained & Rinsed
- 2 Cherry Tomatoes
- 2 Cloves Garlic
- 2 Tablespoons Water
- 2 Teaspoon Honey, Raw
- Black Pepper to Taste
- Pinch Cayenne Pepper

Directions:

1. Mix all of your ingredients in a food processor, and blend until it's smooth.
2. Cover, and place in your fridge before you serve.

Nutritional Info: ‖ Calories: 166 ‖ Protein: 9.4 Grams ‖ Fat: 0.6 Grams ‖ Carbohydrates: 34.2 Grams

Spicy Roasted chickpeas
Time To Prepare: ten minutes
Time to Cook: forty minutes
Yield: Servings 6
Ingredients:

- ¼ teaspoon of cayenne pepper
- 1 teaspoon of paprika
- 1 teaspoon of turmeric
- 2 (fifteen ounce) cans of chickpeas, drained and washed
- 2 teaspoons of coconut oil, melted

Directions:

1. Set the oven to 425°F.
2. Coat a baking sheet using a paper towels, then put the chickpeas on them and use more paper towels to take off the surplus water in the chickpeas. Remove all of the paper towels.
3. Place the oil and spices to the chickpeas and mix thoroughly.
4. Roast your chickpeas for forty minutes, stirring every ten minutes.
5. Once the chickpeas are done, take it off from the oven and let fully cool.

Nutritional Info: ‖ Total Carbohydrates: 19g ‖ Fiber: 6g ‖ Net Carbohydrates: ‖ Protein: 7g ‖ Total Fat: 4g ‖ Calories: 138

Sweet Potato Muffins
Time To Prepare: fifteen minutes
Time to Cook: 20-twenty-five minutes
Yield: Servings 12
Ingredients:

- ¼ Cup Almond Butter

- ¼ Teaspoon Sea Salt
- ½ Teaspoon Baking Soda
- 1 ½ Cups Rolled Oats
- 1 Cup Almond Milk
- 1 Cup Sweet Potato, Cooked & Pureed
- 1 Egg
- 1 Teaspoon Baking Powder
- 1 Teaspoon Ground Cinnamon
- 1 Teaspoon Vanilla Extract, Pure
- 1/3 Cup Coconut Sugar
- 2 Tablespoons Olive Oil

Directions:

1. Begin by heating the oven to 375.
2. Coat your muffin tin with liners, and get out a food processor.
3. Pulse your oats until it forms a course flour. Move it to a small container before setting it to the side.
4. Put in all of your ingredients apart from for the oat flour, blending until the desired smoothness is achieved.
5. Slowly put in in your oat flour, pulsing until it's well blended.
6. Cut between your cupcake liners, and bake for about twenty minutes. Let them cool for minimum five minutes before you serve.

Nutritional Info: ‖ Calories: 143 ‖ Protein: 4 Grams ‖ Fat: 7 Grams ‖ Carbohydrates: 12 Grams

Sweet Sunup Seeds
Time To Prepare: five minutes
Time to Cook: 60 minutes
Yield: Servings 8
Ingredients:

- ¼-cup pure maple syrup
- ¼-cup sunflower oil
- ¼-sesame seeds
- ⅓ -cup honey
- ½-cup flaxseed
- 1-cup dried cranberries

- 1-cup raw pumpkin seeds
- 1-tsp vanilla extract
- 3-tsp cinnamon
- 4-cups rolled oats

Directions:

1. Preheat your oven to 350°F. Prepare two units of baking sheets by lining them using parchment paper.
2. In a large-sized mixing container, mix the rolled oats, pumpkin seeds, flaxseed, sesame seeds, and cinnamon. Mix gently until meticulously blended.
3. Pour all the liquid ingredients into the mixture and stir until mixed well.
4. On the baking sheets, spread the mixture uniformly. Place the sheets in your oven. Cook for minimum an hour. While baking, stir the mixture every quarter of an hour to achieve uniform color on its surfaces.
5. Take away the sheets from the oven. Allow cooling completely. Put in the cup of dried cranberries, and mix thoroughly.
6. Store the granola in an airtight container to maintain its freshness and crunchiness.

Nutritional Info: ‖ Calories: 189 ‖ Fat: 6.3g ‖ Protein: 9.4g ‖ Sodium: 5mg ‖ Total Carbohydrates: 27.6g ‖ Fiber: 4g ‖ Net Carbohydrates: 23.6g

Tangy Turmeric Flavored Florets
Time To Prepare: ten minutes
Time to Cook: 55 minutes
Yield: Servings 1
Ingredients:

- 1-head cauliflower, chopped into florets
- 1-Tbsp olive oil
- 1-Tbsp turmeric
- A dash of salt
- A pinch of cumin

Directions:

1. Set the oven to 400°F.
2. Combine all ingredients in a baking pan. Mix thoroughly until meticulously blended.
3. Cover the pan using foil. Roast for forty minutes. Take away the foil cover and roast additionally for fifteen minutes.

Nutritional Info: ‖ Calories: 90 ‖ Fat: 3g ‖ Protein: 4.5g ‖ Sodium: 87mg ‖ Total Carbohydrates: 16.2g ‖ Fiber: 5g ‖ Net Carbohydrates: 11.2g

Toasted Pumpkin Seeds
Time To Prepare: *five minutes*
Time to Cook: thirty minutes
Yield: Servings 2-4
Ingredients:

- ½ teaspoon extra virgin olive oil
- 1 teaspoon salt
- 1 to 2 cups pumpkin seeds
- Sea salt
- Water

Directions:

1. Put seeds in a deep cooking pan and cover with water. Put in salt.
2. Bring it to its boiling point and boil for about ten minutes.
3. Simmer uncovered for ten more minutes. This makes the seeds very crunchy when baked. Drain the seeds and pat dry using a paper towel.
4. Coat a baking sheet using parchment paper and spread out the seeds in a single layer.
5. Sprinkle with salt, then bake in an oven at 325F for minimum ten minutes, stirring midway through.
6. Cool, then store in an airtight container.

Nutritional Info: ‖ Calories: 192 kcal ‖ Protein: 10.41 g ‖ Fat: 16.23 g ‖ Carbohydrates: 4.34 g

Tofu Pudding
Time To Prepare: *ten minutes*
Time to Cook: *0 minutes*

Yield: Servings 4
Ingredients:

- 1 cup strawberries
- 1 teaspoon honey
- 1 teaspoon pumpkin pie spice
- 1 teaspoon vanilla
- 12 ounces silken tofu, softened and well-drained
- 2 scoops of Protein powder
- 3/4 cup blueberries
- 4 almonds
- Fresh mint leaves

Directions:

1. Combine the tofu and Protein powder in a blender until thoroughly combined.
2. Put in the blueberries, strawberries, honey, pumpkin pie spice, and vanilla. Blend until the desired smoothness is achieved.
3. Cover and put on the refrigerator to chill for minimum 2 hours.
4. Ladle into four dessert bowls and top with an almond and a mint leaf before you serve.

Nutritional Info: ‖ Calories: 371 kcal ‖ Protein: 23.31 g ‖ Fat: 21.1 g ‖ Carbohydrates: 27.17 g

Turmeric Chickpea Cakes
Time To Prepare: twenty minutes
Time to Cook: thirty minutes
Yield: Servings 8
Ingredients:

- ½ cup fresh parsley, minced
- 1 teaspoon cayenne pepper, to taste (not necessary)
- 1 teaspoon salt or to taste
- 2 cans (15oz.) chickpeas, washed, drained
- 2 small onions, minced
- 2 teaspoons turmeric powder
- 4 cloves garlic, minced
- 4 tablespoons cornstarch

- 8-10 tablespoons chickpea flour
- Avocado dipping sauce to serve
- Freshly ground pepper to taste
- Grapeseed oil to fry

Directions:

1. Put a frying pan on moderate heat. Put in a little oil. When the oil is heated, put onion and garlic and sauté until translucent. Remove the heat and cool to room temperature.
2. Put in chickpeas into the food processor container and pulse until very finely chopped.
3. Put in the onion mixture, salt, pepper, cayenne pepper, and turmeric powder and pulse again until well blended.
4. Move into a container. Put in parsley and mix thoroughly.
5. Make small balls of the mixture (of approximately 1 inch diameter) and mould into patties. Put chickpea flour on a plate.
6. Put a nonstick pan on moderate heat. Put in a little oil and swirl the pan so that the oil spreads.
7. Immerse the patties in the chickpea flour and place a few on the pan. Cook in batches.
8. Cook until the underside is golden brown. Flip then cook the other side till it's golden brown.
9. Repeat steps 6-8 to fry the rest of the patties.
10. Serve with avocado dipping sauce.

Nutritional Info: ‖ Calories: 154 kcal ‖ Protein: 7.32 g ‖ Fat: 2.85 g ‖ Carbohydrates: 25.43 g

Turmeric Coconut Flour Muffins
Time To Prepare: *five minutes*
Time to Cook: twenty-five minutes
Yield: Servings 8
Ingredients:

- ½ cup Unsweetened coconut milk
- ½ tsp. Baking soda
- ½ tsp. Ginger powder
- ¾ cup & 2 tbsp. Coconut flour
- 1 tsp. Vanilla extract

- 1/3 cup Maple syrup
- 2 tsp. Turmeric
- 6 big Whole eggs
- Pepper and salt

Directions:

1. Preheat your oven to 350°F.
2. Coat 8 muffin tins with 8 muffin liners.
3. Whisk eggs, maple syrup, milk, and vanilla extract in a mixing container until the egg begins to make bubbles.
4. In a different container, combine the coconut flour, turmeric powder, pepper, baking soda, ginger powder, and salt.
5. Place the dry mixture into the wet mixture then stir until it's all mixed and thick.
6. Ladle out the batter into prepared muffin tins.
7. Leave to bake for about twenty-five minutes or until it looked golden.
8. Allow the muffins cool for a couple of minutes before transferring them to a rack.

Nutritional Info: ‖ Calories: 143 kcal ‖ Protein: 6.18 g ‖ Fat: 8 g ‖ Carbohydrates: 11.8 g

Turmeric Gummies
Time To Prepare: five minutes
Time to Cook: 4 hours and ten minutes
Yield: Servings 4
Ingredients:

- ¼ tsp. Ground pepper
- 1 tsp. Ground turmeric
- 3 ½ cups Water
- 6 tbsp. Maple syrup
- 8 tbsp. Unflavored gelatin powder

Directions:

1. Combine the ground turmeric, maple syrup, and water in a pot set on moderate heat. Stir continuously for five minutes before

removing from heat and pouring in the gelatin powder. Stir using a wooden spoon to dissolve the gelatin.

2. Put back the pan on the heat and stir for another two minutes.

3. Remove the heat and take the mixture to a deep container that you will seal using plastic wrapimmediately after.

4. Place in your fridge the mixture for approximately 4 hours.

5. It must be firm now, cut it into little squares, and serve or store.

Nutritional Info: ‖ Calories: 123 kcal ‖ Protein: 2.15 g ‖ Fat: 1.56 g ‖ Carbohydrates: 25.67 g

Soups and Stews
Anti-inflammatory Spring Pea Soup
Time To Prepare:five minutes
Time to Cook: fifteen minutes
Yield: Servings 6
Ingredients:

- ½ tsp. Black pepper powder
- ½ tsp. ground cumin
- 1 liter Vegetable stock
- 1 medium Chopped onion
- 2 tbsp. Coconut oil
- 2 tsp. Celtic sea salt
- 700 g. Fresh peas
- Chopped flat-leaf parsley
- Chopped mint leaves
- Fresh lemon juice
- Grated nutmeg
- Toasted sunflower seeds

Directions:

1. Warm the coconut oil in a pan set on moderate heat.

2. Mix in onions and stir fry for approximately five minutes.

3. Put in the stock and raise the heat. Throw in fresh peas and cook for five minutes. If you're using frozen peas, it should take half the time.

4. Pour in the lemon juice, salt, pepper, herbs, and spices. Stirring continuously

5. Remove the heat and allow it to cool before running it through a food processor to whatever consistency you prefer.
6. Serve with sunflower seed sprinkles and mint or parsley leaves.
7. Enjoy!

Nutritional Info: Calories: 115 kcal ‖ Protein: 5 g ‖ Fat: 5.91 g ‖ Carbohydrates: 11.8 g

Anti-Inflammatory Sweet Potato Soup
Time To Prepare: twenty minutes
Time to Cook: thirty minutes
Yield: Servings 8
Ingredients:

- 1 13.66-ounce can lite coconut milk
- 1 big zucchini, cut width-wise
- 1 garlic clove
- 1 liter low-sodium vegetable stock
- 1 tablespoon sweet yellow curry powder
- 1 teaspoon black pepper
- 1 teaspoon cayenne pepper
- 1 teaspoon turmeric
- 1 white onion
- 2 moderate-sized white potatoes,
- 3 moderate-sized sweet potatoes,
- 3/4 tablespoons salt
- 4 cups of hot water
- 4 tablespoons olive oil
- A pinch of cinnamon
- A pinch of cloves

Directions:

1. Prepare every one of your vegetables by cutting, cleaning & cubing. Put in a safe spot.
2. To a large pot, include 4 tablespoons of additional virgin olive oil. Allow it to heat up swiftly; at that point, include your white onion. Allow it to sweat for minimum five minutes on low warmth.

3. Put in all your flavoring & garlic. Give it a decent mix; at that point, including the potatoes.

4. Allow these cook on moderate heat for around five minutes to get a pleasant darker shading. Continue blending to abstain from consuming.

5. Put in your stalk & water, warm it to the point of boiling & then stew for around 20-twenty-five minutes. Part of the way through the stewing procedure, include your zucchini.

6. After 20-twenty-five minutes, include your coconut milk. Before pouring the soup to the blender, do a fork content to guarantee your potatoes are cooked.

7. Use your blender to purée the soup. Embellishment with lemon juice, dark pepper & herbs & flavors of your preference.

Nutritional Info: Calories: 281 kcal ‖ Protein: 4.1 g ‖ Fat: 20.22 g ‖ Carbohydrates: 23.8 g

Bacon & Cheese Soup
Time To Prepare: fifteen minutes
Time to Cook: forty minutes
Yield: Servings 6
Ingredients:

- ½ cup sour cream, for serving
- ½ teaspoon cumin
- ½ teaspoon onion powder
- ½ teaspoon paprika
- 1 cup heavy cream
- 1 cup shredded cheddar cheese
- 1 pound of lean ground beef
- 1 tablespoon coconut oil, for cooking
- 1 teaspoon garlic powder
- 1 yellow onion, chopped
- 6 cups beef broth
- 6 slices uncured bacon

Directions:

1. Put in the coconut oil to a frying pan and cook the bacon until

crunchy. Allow the bacon to cool and cut into little pieces. Set aside.

2. Once cooked, put in the lean ground beef to the same frying pan with the bacon fat and cook until browned.

3. Put in the onions and cook for an extra two to three minutes.

4. Put in all the ingredients minus the bacon, heavy cream, sour cream and cheese to a stockpot and stir. Cook for about twenty-five minutes.

5. Warm the heavy cream, and then put in the warmed cream and cheese and serve with the bacon and a spoonful of sour cream.

Nutritional Info: Calories: 498 ‖ Carbohydrates: 5g ‖ Fiber: 1g Net ‖ Carbohydrates: 4g ‖ Fat: 34g ‖ Protein: 41g

Chapter Four

WHAT IS THE RIGHT DIET FOR RHEUMATISM?

*A*nyone who suffers from rheumatism can alleviate the symptoms with a suitable diet. Doctors assume that it is even possible to have a positive influence on the intake of medication. Above all, it is important to reduce the consumption of meat and sausage. Many nutrition experts also recommend a plant-based diet. It should be supplemented with dairy products and fish, with the low-fat variants being preferred. The cause is thought to be that you consume less arachidonic acid through such foods. It has the reputation of promoting inflammation in the body and thus gives your rheumatism a direct boost. Arachidonic acid is a fatty acid, it is mainly found in fatty dairy products and meat. The situation is different for plant-based foods; they do not contain these fatty acids or only to a very limited extent. Seafood or fish are also not entirely free of arachidonic acid. At the same time, however, they also have a high content of fatty acids with a positive influence, such as the important omega-3 fatty acids. Vegetable oils also contain fatty acids, and they are also generally ascribed a positive effect.

The situation is similar with dairy products. Arachidonic acid can also be found in it, but milk and its by-products are rich in protein and calcium. Calcium is an important part of the bones, it strengthens them and helps prevent osteoporosis. In order to use the positive properties of dairy products as much as possible, rheumatism sufferers should mainly eat low-fat milk and dairy products because they contain a small proportion of the inflammation-promoting fatty acids. Every patient must know that a suitable diet can alleviate the symptoms. Nevertheless, you should always seek professional treatment from a doctor and also take the recommended medication. Even with a very well balanced diet, the inflammatory processes in the body can only be controlled and positively influenced to a certain extent. There is a lot you can do to make yourself better yourself, but you should definitely not go without the care of your doctor. So let your doctor know that you are changing your diet and let them give you the best tips to do so. In this way you yourself contribute to a positive course of your illness. Now that you have got a first insight into the right diet for rheumatism, in the following paragraph we give you a few tips on how you can design your menu in the future.

The best tips for proper nutrition in everyday life

As a rheumatoid patient, you probably have a keen interest in eating yourself in a way that is good for yourself. Even so, it can be difficult to change your diet so that it has a positive effect on your rheumatism. For many patients it is difficult to get used to a completely new form of diet overnight. This is even more true if you do not feel the positive influence immediately because the body does not react within a few days. It is far too easy to get discouraged and stop eating a diet suitable for rheumatism, even though you were actually on the right track.

In such cases, perseverance is very helpful. Remember that your body needs a few days to adjust to the changed supply of nutrients. This is even more true when you want to cut down on certain harmful fatty acids in the body, thereby reducing the potential for inflammation. So give yourself and your body the necessary time and rest so that it slowly gets used to your rheumatic-appropriate diet. Also try not to change everything immediately and in the first week, but rather take the individual steps with a time delay. You may find it easier to start with one step for two weeks and then move on to the next step for another two weeks. Keep in mind that it will take some time to get used to the change in your diet and to fully adjust to it. So take the necessary rest and patience, because you will soon find that it is worthwhile and that your symptoms are slowly improving a little. So what general nutrition tips are there for rheumatism patients, and how can you incorporate them into your everyday life? If you take a closer look, you will find that most of the tips are not that different from the general recommendations for healthy eating.

1. Eliminate fat from your diet

The first tip is especially difficult for you if you like to eat high in fat. If possible, avoid all high-fat foods of animal origin. This mainly means lard, egg yolks, butter, cream, egg yolks and sausage and cheese with a high fat content. Remember that you do not have to eliminate these foods from your menu! Opt for the low-fat variants or alternatives with a low fat content. This will reduce the intake of harmful fatty acids. By the way, with a low-fat diet you also help to lose one or two kilograms of excess weight. This is particularly useful because your joints, which are already affected, are even more stressed by being overweight. If you manage to lose weight, you will also relieve your joints.

2. Cut down on meat and sausage

It will also have a very beneficial effect if you significantly reduce the consumption of sausage and meat. Try to eat meat and sausage in all variations no more than twice a week. Again, if you eat meat or sausage, remember to resort to the low-fat alternatives. This change not only reduces the amount of harmful fatty acids in your body. At the same time, you have the option of further reducing the intake of calories, which makes it easier to lose weight.

3. Fruits and vegetables are healthy and delicious

You probably know the rules of eating five servings of fruit and vegetables a day. One serving is as much as you can hold in one hand. So it's the equivalent of a banana, an apple, or as many grapes as you can pick up in one hand. Which types of fruit or which vegetables you eat play a subordinate role. Decide on the varieties that you like. Above all, ensure that there is a change in the menu so that it doesn't get boring. You are also welcome to use the cooked variants, because cooked fruit and vegetables are often easier for the body to process and use. Canned fruit or vegetables are not very suitable for your rheumatic diet. Of course, they can of course also be consumed once in an emergency, but you should usually ensure that the goods are fresh. If you can, you are happy to use food from the region, because they have a shorter transport route and are therefore usually fresher. Organic fruit or vegetables are also recommended if you have the opportunity to buy.

4. Fish should be on the table regularly

Tip number four may be difficult to implement for many people. Make an effort to eat fish twice a week. This can be salmon, mackerel or herring, for example. You can combine fish very well with rice, pasta or potatoes and conjure up a new dish for every day of the week. Of course you can also try the vegetarian options, but fish contains valuable fatty acids and is therefore very good for the body.

5. Healthy fat is allowed

As you already know, you should aim for a low-fat diet. However, there are some oils that are very rich in the important omega-3 fatty acids and vitamin E. Vitamin E in particular protects your joints from wear and tear and should therefore be taken in sufficient quantities. Soybean oil, walnut oil, rapeseed or linseed oil are rich in vitamin E. Nuts are also very healthy and contain important fatty acids. Eat them straight or use them as a side dish in muesli or in a salad. Make sure you only consume a few nuts, because although they are very healthy, they are also high in calories.

With these five tips, you should be able to switch to a healthy diet step by step in order to improve your rheumatism. In the next chapter we will deal intensively with a gift from nature that is a little underestimated in a healthy diet. Spices and herbs have an enormous influence on our organism. Use the little treasures with their positive influences and always round off your meals with the right spices. By the way, you trigger anti-inflammatory processes in the body that can alleviate your symptoms without you having to do more than spice it up properly.

HOW TO HARNESS THE POWER OF SPICES

You can get many of the herbs and spices listed below when shopping in a well-stocked supermarket or in a drugstore with a grocery department. If possible, make sure that the spices are of good organic quality. You will feel it in the intense taste and simply eat with a better feeling. By the way, it is by no means just the exotic spices that are said to have anti-inflammatory effects. There are also delicious ingredients from the region that can have a positive effect on your rheumatism with their ingredients.

Turmeric - also known as turmeric - tops the list of spices with anti-inflammatory properties. Popular in Indian dishes and especially in all kinds of curry, turmeric can also be added to many other dishes. Curcuma contains curcumin, which can reduce inflammation.

Cumin actually comes from oriental cuisine and is often used there to flavor falafel and similar dishes. Cumin tastes a bit spicy and a bit fruity with a sharp note. For example, mix a little cumin with coriander and oil and stir the mixture with a little oil to season your dishes.

In Chinese and Ayurvedic cuisine, ginger is often used for cooking. The yellow tuber is rich in essential oils and contains antioxidants. They have a neutralizing effect on free radicals in the body, which can promote the development of inflammation.

Cinnamon also has an anti-inflammatory effect. Secondary plant substances are contained in cinnamon, and cinnamon is said to have a lowering effect on the cholesterol level and blood sugar.

If you like chili, you will surely be happy that the hot pods can stimulate blood circulation and thus reduce inflammation. Local onions or garlic are also said to be rich in anti-inflammatory ingredients, with sulfur compounds being the cause. They can disinfect and have an antibacterial effect. Perhaps you combine these spices with paprika, which should be rich in antioxidants and which should therefore have an anti-inflammatory effect on the organism.

Unfortunately, there are only a few studies that substantiate the positive effects of spices and herbs on diseases from a medical point of view. However, Ayurvedic cuisine in particular likes to work with herbs a lot. The art of Ayurveda is many 1,000 years old, and countless treatments and recommendations for the relief of complaints have their origins here. It can therefore be assumed that spices can certainly contribute to your healthy eating. Take this opportunity and add a few recommendations to your repertoire of herbs and spices in the kitchen. Feel free to try out which spices you like with which dishes. Perhaps this creates one or the other creation with a slight touch of oriental or Indian cuisine that you previously did not think possible. Your health could thank you, because anti-inflammatory ingredients in your food can ultimately help your rheumatism get a little better and prevent your symptoms from getting worse. In the next chapter you will find out what else you need to know about anti-inflammatory nutrition.

WHY IS ARTICULAR CARTILAGE SO IMPORTANT?

Cartilage is found wherever two bones come into contact when moving. It is a flexible connection between two bones and ensures that we can move our joints at all. If there is a misalignment such as X or O legs or heavy loads such as being overweight, the cartilage is affected, cracks and frayed. In the course of osteoarthritis, the cartilage coating can be completely lost. The bones begin to rub against each other and are forced to reshape. The skin around the joint turns red and there is swelling. Strong pain restricts those affected more and more in their movement.

WHAT ROLE DOES SYNOVIAL FLUID PLAY?

Our cartilage tissue is extremely sensitive because, unlike many other parts of the body, it is not covered by blood vessels. Vital nutrients have to get to the necessary places via the synovial fluid. The so-called synovial fluid is formed by the synovial membrane. Regular movement distributes the fluid in the cartilage so that it remains supple and can regenerate. At the same time, the synovial fluid acts as a buffer and supports the cartilage in cushioning impacts on the joint. With osteoarthritis these processes are disturbed. The synovial fluid has a different consistency; it is more fluid than in a healthy joint. As a result, it is distributed faster, but it also loses its effect as a buffer.

CAUGHT IN A VICIOUS CIRCLE

The fact that those affected no longer see themselves able to move leads to the spread of inflammation because important nutrients are no longer transported to the joints. The lack of movement increases the pain more and more. It is therefore important not to take it easy in spite of the pain, but to do sports such as swimming, cycling or hiking that do not put too much strain on the joint.

SYMPTOMS

The consequences and symptoms are just as varied as the forms of osteoarthritis that occur. While one patient does not feel the effects of his illness until very late, another complains early on of severe symptoms. Typical symptoms of osteoarthritis are:
- Joint stiffeners
- Capsular ligament injuries
- Deformities
- instability of the joint
- flare-ups
- Formation of effusions
- swelling

In addition, many sufferers complain of severe pain in an advanced stage, which in turn can be divided into three categories:

Start-up pain: As the name suggests, this pain occurs mainly at the beginning of a movement. The joint is insufficiently lubricated when it is resting and it takes some time for the body to produce enough synovial fluid through movement so that the bone surfaces no longer rub against each other.

Fatigue or exertion pain: With this form of pain, the pain arises directly in the joint due to increasing abrasion of the cartilage layer. The body releases enzymes to break down tissue and cell debris, but also attacks the already damaged cartilage. As a result, an inflammatory reaction occurs in the joint, causing the pain. As the disease progresses, this pain continues to increase.

Pain at rest: Pain at rest occurs in the course of what is known as "activated osteoarthritis" when an inflammatory process is already underway in the joint. It can be felt even when the joint is not moved.

STAGES OF OSTEOARTHRITIS

Osteoarthritis is a gradual process that can be divided into different stages. The joints often wear out for many years before symptoms can be noticed. Especially at the beginning, the symptoms are so weak that they are not recognized by affected people or only recognized very late. However, early diagnosis and appropriate treatment can significantly slow the course of osteoarthritis. In principle, osteoarthritis can be divided into two stages:

First stage (primary osteoarthritis): In the first stage of the disease, the layers of cartilage fray and become inflamed. Primary osteoarthritis can only be seen on the X-ray.

Second stage (secondary osteoarthritis): If the cartilage is further affected, it continues to wear out until it is completely rubbed off in the second and last stage of osteoarthritis and the bones rub against each other. As an emergency reaction of the body, excesses or stiffening develop on the joints, which are also easily recognizable from the outside. If the osteoarthritis remains untreated, the bone is increasingly destroyed. This stage can be recognized by a missing joint space and insufficient mobility of the joint.

Intermediate stage:
There may be many years between the first and second stages of osteoarthritis, so that most of those affected are in an intermediate stage. Often there is already no cartilage left in some parts of the joint, so that hardening and expansion form in the bone.

WHICH JOINTS ARE AFFECTED?

Many people associate osteoarthritis with the knees, as this is where the disease is most common. However, this does not mean that other joints cannot be affected as well. Pain in the following joints can indicate an early stage of osteoarthritis:

Hands: This form of osteoarthritis is often only recognized late. Typical symptoms are stiff, swollen fingers that are restricted in their mobility. Swollen, reddened or even over-heated joints indicate active osteoarthritis. In the course of the disease, additional thickenings can develop on the finger joints, from which a gelatinous liquid oozes. Bony thickenings on the right and left of the joints are also typical for the advanced course of this form of osteoarthritis. Osteoarthritis in the joints of the hands and fingers is up to ten times as common in menopausal women than in men. It is therefore assumed that changes in the hormonal balance are responsible for the development of this form of osteoarthritis. Genetics also seem to have an impact. Women whose relatives also suffer from osteoarthritis are more likely to develop osteoarthritis of the fingers and wrists over the course of their lives.

Hip: Hip osteoarthritis is one of the most common forms of osteoarthritis caused by obesity, inflammatory joint diseases or misalignments such as X and O legs. The first signs of joint wear and tear are hip pain when running and especially when climbing stairs. However, a reliable diagnosis can only be given by an examination of the hip by the doctor.

Knee: Knee osteoarthritis, also known as osteoarthritis of the knee, is an increasing wear and tear on the knee joints. Here, too, pain is the first symptom of the disease and should be clarified by a doctor as early as possible. Untreated osteoarthritis of the knee can ultimately even lead to the joints stiffening and the affected person having to rely on an operation and the use of an artificial knee joint.

Toes: With osteoarthritis in the toes, basically only one toe is meant. In the so-called hallux rigidus, the joint of the big toe becomes inflamed and the joint space narrows. Hallux rigidus can be treated quite well in the early stages. With insoles, hyaluronic acid or cortisone injections and special insoles, the progression of the disease can be slowed down so much that further consequences can be largely prevented. Only an operation to relieve the pain in the joint can often only help in the late stages. Hallux rigidus can be recognized by the stabbing pain when walking and painful water retention in the bones under the joint surface.

If one of these joints is affected, the risk of developing osteoarthritis in other areas increases. After all, the inflammatory processes do not have a targeted effect, but are distributed throughout the body.

How the right diet can help with osteoarthritis

The right diet helps against osteoarthritis in many ways. A combination of a healthy BMI and a balanced diet relieves the joints and supplies the cartilage and bones with sufficient nutrients. The consumption of certain foods, on the other hand, favors inflammatory processes in the body and contributes to the development of obesity. The following section reveals which foods should be avoided in osteoarthritis, which nutrients should be consumed and which foods are best for treating osteoarthritis.

Weight reduction:
Patients with osteoarthritis are often told by their doctor that the first step should be to lose weight. Why this is so can be summed up in one sentence: Knees and hip joints no longer have to carry such a heavy load and the body no longer has to fight against so many inflammatory processes. But not only the reduced weight has a positive effect on osteoarthritis. The improved metabolism also provides relief from osteoarthritis by reducing the increased blood sugar and fat values.

... through fasting cures:
Fasting cures, i.e. avoiding solid and high-calorie food, are recommended as an introduction to behavior change. The body is dependent on its own reserves, there is rapid weight loss and the basic attitude towards food intake changes. After the fasting days, a balanced diet should be aimed for, which further promotes weight loss in a gentle way.

... through intermediate fasting:
Intermittent fasting is also particularly popular because, in contrast to therapeutic fasting, it is much easier to implement and can be sustained over a longer period of time. Here phases of food intake alternate with phases of fasting. Solid food and high-calorie drinks should be avoided for a total of 16 hours at a time. This is followed by a time window of 8 hours in which you can eat up to three times. It should be noted that the 16 hours are always in a time window in which fasting is easy, because 8 hours of it are overslept anyway. After a short period of change, the body gets used to the extended fasting period and the feeling of hunger decreases.

... through an alkaline diet:
Many patients swear by an alkaline diet for osteoarthritis, but does this

type of diet actually help with weight loss? The aim is to achieve a balanced acid-base ratio and thus an optimal PH value in the body through the choice of food. If the acid content in the blood is too high, it flows only slowly and can no longer transport inflammation-promoting substances as effectively. Since a lot of fruit and vegetables are consumed in the alkaline diet, there is usually a rapid weight reduction here too. In addition, the basic foods are often among those that have a positive effect against osteoarthritis.

AFTERWORD

Set goals: Break your goals down into lots of small goals and reward yourself regularly. This is the only way to maintain motivation over the long term. However, the rewards shouldn't consist of high-calorie foods, but rather material things. Make a list of things that you always wanted to treat yourself to and tick off a point after each goal you achieved.

Establish a routine: make a schedule of when to eat, when to buy the healthy meals, when to prepare them and then stick to it meticulously. Establish a routine by combining the practical with the useful. You pass a supermarket after work? Then take this opportunity to go shopping. Once you are in the cozy home, it is difficult to step outside the front door again and the probability is higher that you will resort to ready-made meals.

Trying out new things: Deliberately engage in new culinary experiments and try foods and dishes that you have never tried before. For example, try out the vegetarian or vegan cuisine for a week and see for yourself that fruit and vegetables alone can satisfy your hunger and still taste very varied and delicious.

Drink a lot: Water is the only food that has a negative energy balance. That means: if you drink a lot of water, you burn additional calories during the day. Many people find it difficult to switch from unsweetened drinks to water at first, which is why certain types of tea are recommended. Green and black tea, for example, stimulate the metabolism and, due to their high caffeine content, are excellent coffee substitutes.

Losing weight together: Losing weight permanently is a challenge that most people find so difficult that in most cases they give up and afterwards put even more pounds on the scales due to the yo-yo effect. On the other hand, those who join forces with others early on and exchange experiences have a greater chance of success, because knowledge is power here too. And it learns from the mistakes of others as well as from its own. Every problem you face while losing weight has already been recognized and solved by others before you. For every stumbling block there is a suitable strategy for you to avoid it.

WHICH NUTRIENTS ARE IMPORTANT IN OSTEOARTHRITIS?: VITAMIN C:

Among other things, this vitamin is said to alleviate pain caused by osteoarthritis. By promoting the so-called collagen synthesis, cartilage tissue is formed more quickly and osteoarthritis is further contained.

Vitamin D:

Often referred to as the sun vitamin, vitamin D can be recharged particularly well on long walks in the fresh air. The immune system is strengthened and inflammation is reduced. A deficiency of this important vitamin, on the other hand, favors the course of osteoarthritis.

Vitamin E:

Vitamin E also relieves pain in many ways and has a positive effect on osteoarthritis. In addition, the formation of arachidonic acid is blocked. The vitamin unfolds its full effect in connection with the absorption of vitamin C. Both vitamins are mainly found in carrots, bell peppers, leafy vegetables such as spinach as well as in citrus and berry fruits.

Manganese:

In order to optimally support the structure of cartilage in the body, the intake of manganese through diet is essential. Manganese helps protect healthy bones and the formation of new connective tissue by increasing the effects of chondroitin and glucosamine.

Zinc:

Zinc also plays an important role in bone maintenance. In addition, it contributes to a good acid-base metabolism and healthy protein synthesis.

Copper:

Copper has an antioxidant and anti-inflammatory effect and is an important component in the prevention and relief of osteoarthritis, which also has a positive effect on the resistance of the connective tissue.

Selenium:

In order for the body to be able to produce sufficient antioxidant enzymes, it needs an adequate supply of selenium. With a balanced selenium balance, this nutrient inhibits the inflammatory activity of the affected joints.

Omega-3 fatty acids:

In contrast to the omega-6 fatty acids, these fatty acids are very important for joint health, because in high doses the omega-3 fatty acids successfully counteract pain and joint inflammation.

Carbohydrates:

Carbohydrates supply the body with energy directly through blood sugar. However, not all carbohydrates are created equal. While sugar, for example, consists of simple carbohydrates and can cause tooth decay and often has a negative effect on body weight, more complex carbohydrates have a positive effect on the intestines and their relatively low calorie content ensures weight reduction. High-fiber foods such as fruits and vegetables are particularly recommended. Potatoes and whole grain products in particular are rich in valuable fiber, fill you up and help the intestines to function properly.

Proteins:

Protein and proteins are often associated with athletes because they are an important building block for the development of muscles and cannot be produced by the body itself. Protein also plays a major role in the formation of important hormones and enzymes that ensure smooth digestion.

Fats:

When it comes to the group of fats, it is also important to differentiate between good and harmful fats. The group of bad fats consists mainly of animal fats such as meat or dairy products. Good fats, on the other hand, include foods that have anti-inflammatory effects. In the case of osteoarthritis, all vitamin E-rich vegetable oils and diet or health margarine are recommended. Olive and rapeseed oil may also be used, as they contain simple unsaturated fatty acids that protect the blood vessels. In principle, fat should only be consumed in moderation, as this nutrient is by far the most energetic and therefore often has a negative effect on body weight.

Bromelain:

Is responsible for healing inflammatory processes and is mainly found in pineapples, bromelain has a pain-relieving effect, boosts the immune system and promotes blood circulation. Healing processes are accelerated and the mobility of the joints is increased. In addition, bromelain gradually reduces the swelling around the joint and is therefore a real miracle cure for osteoarthritis.

Chondroitin sulfate:

Obtained from bovine cartilage, this component of the cartilage tissue promotes the body's natural water retention and contributes to the development of new cartilage substance. In addition, chondroitin sulfate helps to regenerate the synovial fluid. However, more than 700 mg per day should not be consumed.

Glucosamine sulfate:

Together with chondroitin sulfate, this nutrient has a pain-relieving effect and is a natural component of the bone and synovial fluid. The glucosamine obtained from cancer shells stimulates the body's own synthesis of cartilage tissue and alleviates inflammation. However, more than 1200mg per day leads to undesirable side effects.

PREFERRED FOODS FOR OSTEOARTHRITIS

There is a whole list of foods that are said to have beneficial effects on joint problems. It is therefore quite possible to specifically support bones and cartilage with the right combination of nutrients. In general, the menu should consist of foods rich in vitamins and low in fat. The micronutrients vitamin E and C as well as zinc, selenium, copper and manganese are particularly important because they intercept free radicals and help reduce oxidative stress. The following section describes the functions of the individual nutrients in more detail.

Salad:

Salad plants such as lettuce, iceberg lettuce, endive, rocket, chicory and lamb's lettuce contain particularly high levels of ß-carotene, which has an antioxidant effect. As a rule of thumb, all types of dark lettuce can be consumed in large quantities without hesitation.

Types of cabbage:

Different types of cabbage such as cauliflower, broccoli, green or red cabbage are excellent sources of glucosinolate. These are plant substances with an antioxidant effect. Broccoli and kale also provide a lot and calcium.

Tuber vegetables:

The tubers include fennel, kohlrabi, and celery. This group supplies the body with numerous phytochemicals and a lot of vitamin C.

Carrots:

As the name suggests, carrots contain a lot of ß-carotene. However, the carrots should not be eaten raw, as the ß-carotene is only available to the body after juicing.

Leek vegetables:

... Like onions or garlic, their sulfur compounds have anti-inflammatory effects and protect the cartilage.

Legumes:

Whether lentils, beans or peas - pulses are protein and fiber suppliers with lots of purines and should therefore be regularly on the menu.

All kinds of fruit:

Despite its high fructose content, fruit is an indispensable part of our diet. It contains a mix of the most important vitamins and many minerals. You can eat it either in solid form or as a juice. The ingredients are retained in both variants. However, you should make sure that fruit juices from the supermarket do not contain any added sugar.

Whole grain products:

Whole grains such as spelled and whole wheat, muesli with no added sugar, brown rice and whole wheat pasta are rich in fiber and ensure a good satiety and a healthy intestinal flora. They also have a positive effect on blood sugar and contain numerous vitamins and minerals such as zinc and copper.

Bone and Cartilage Broth:

What sounds repulsive at first glance turns out to be a centuries-old remedy for joint problems, which is mainly used in naturopathy.

Mineral water:

As the only food that consumes more calories during processing than it absorbs, mineral water is a real miracle cure for weight loss, and it also contains plenty of calcium for the bones.

FOOD TO AVOID IN OSTEOARTHRITIS

Since our diet has a significant influence on the inflammatory processes in the body, foods that promote the development of inflammation should be avoided in osteoarthritis. The group of foods that promote inflammation include:

White flour products:
Like white bread, toasted bread and peeled rice, the body quickly converts them into sugar and must always be replaced with whole grain products.

Processed potato products:
French fries, potato pancakes and co. dripping with fat and deep-fried in oils that contain inflammatory omega-6 fatty acids. You should definitely keep your hands off these products.

Dairy products:
High-fat dairy products such as full-fat milk, camembert and semi-hard cheese contain many inflammatory fats.

The situation is similar with sweetened milk products such as fruit yoghurt, fruit buttermilk or fruit quark. Mix your unsweetened dairy products yourself with some fresh fruit to achieve the sweetness you want.

High-fat meat:
Meat and high-fat sausage products such as meat loaf, bacon, salami, liver sausage support the inflammatory processes in the body and damage the joints. Pork and lard also contain many of the inflammatory arachidonic acids.

Sugar:
Industrially produced white sugar should be avoided.

Animal fat:
Animal fats in sausage or meat products add arachidonic acid to the body, while inflammatory messengers are formed in the body from omega-6 fatty acids. For this reason, cheese, butter, milk and eggs should also be avoided.

Stay away from alcohol and caffeine:
It is well known that water and tea have a very positive effect on health. Since it will be extremely difficult for many to completely avoid these two foods, at least moderate consumption is advisable.

These foods should only be consumed occasionally
Nightshade family:
Eggplants, tomatoes, peppers, potatoes and asparagus belong to the group of the post-shade plants. For the vast majority of patients, these plants should be consumed without hesitation, but for a few people they can also worsen the joint inflammation. Here it is important to test the tolerance or rather seldom strike right at the beginning.

Low fat dairy products:

Reduced-fat milk, natural yoghurt or cream cheese, as well as reduced-fat cheese in general, Harz cheese, sour cream or buttermilk often only contain little arachidonic acid and therefore do not have as inflammation-promoting effects as full-fat products, but contain a similar amount of protein, zinc and calcium.

Beef:
Compared to other meats such as pork, beef is less inflammatory because it contains lower amounts of arachidonic acid and is often low in fat.

Poultry:
For people with osteoarthritis who are reluctant to go without meat, poultry meat is probably the best alternative because it has little fat and a lot of healthy protein.

Lean meat and lean sausages:
The high protein content and low concentration of arachidonic acid are also considered to be well suited for occasional consumption in the case of beef fillet and sliced turkey breast.

Rapeseed, linseed and olive oil:
Due to their extremely high fat content, oils should generally be consumed with caution. However, some varieties contain less harmful omega-3 fatty acids and vitamins, so they can be consumed occasionally without concern.

Walnuts:
Because of their alpha-linolenic acid and their high content of omega-3 fatty acids, walnuts are considered anti-inflammatory and have even been shown to improve the body's fat levels. However, due to their extremely high calorie density, walnuts should be consumed in small quantities.

Nuts and seeds in general:
Other types of nuts such as hazelnuts, Brazil nuts, cashews, flax seeds and pumpkin seeds also contain valuable fatty acids, but have a similar number of calories, so that a maximum of a handful of nuts a day is completely sufficient.